"With clarity and keen insight, Drs. Olsen and Dr. Sharfstein trace the opioid overdose epidemic back to its roots, and lay out the steps that every community needs to take going forward to prevent overdoses and save lives. *The Opioid Epidemic* is absolutely essential reading for those who are just getting up to speed on this national health crisis and for seasoned public health and policy professionals alike."

—Nicole Alexander-Scott, Commissioner of Health for Rhode Island and President, Association of State and Territorial Health Officials

"Understanding the addiction epidemic in the US today is a daunting task. This is a complex issue crossing many disciplines—health services, criminal justice, law enforcement, and family systems. This book is excellent in offering the most up-to-date orientation of the history of the disease, laws, causes, treatment, and, most of all, hope. I wish this book had been available when my son was struggling for his life. A must read for those who suffer and those who love them. Great primer for medical professionals, law enforcement and any others who want to be part of the solution of healing and hope."

Barbara Allen, Executive Director and Founder, James Place and Chair, Howard County Opioid Council

"As two of the most distinguished experts on addiction and the opioid epidemic, Drs. Olsen and Sharfstein have written a definitive guide to understanding the epidemic and arming readers with information backed by science and evidence to help themselves, their loved ones, and their communities."

Michael Botticelli, Executive Director, Grayken Center for Addiction Medicine and former Director, White House Office of National Drug Control Policy

"This is a one-of-a-kind, comprehensive review of everything to know about the opioid epidemic. Drs. Olsen and Sharfstein have made complex issues accessible and digestible to the reader. This book should be read by everyone involved in the opioid epidemic— especially patients, family members, health care providers, and policy makers."

—Chinazo Cunningham, Addiction Medicine Physician, Albert Einstein School of Medicine

"Years into our nation's lethal and unrelenting opioid epidemic, we are still missing a level-setting work that equips us with the language, concepts, science, and tools to truly tackle the crisis together. Drs. Olsen and Sharfstein have given us just that: an accessible and compelling account of the opioid epidemic in all of its dimensions, including the best path out of it. It should be required reading for everyone contending with the crisis, in other words, for all of us."
—**Brandon del Pozo, Chief of Police, Burlington, Vermont**

"In highlighting the worst public health disaster facing Americans in a generation, Olsen and Sharfstein methodically provide riveting insights in a relentlessly logical manner. The book is the most comprehensive and insightful look at the opioid crisis from its origins to what it will take to solve this epidemic, written in a clear and concise manner. A must read for everyone."
—**Rahul Gupta, Former Commissioner and**
State Health Officer for West Virginia

"In this pragmatic and accessible book Drs. Olsen and Sharfstein unrelentingly explain and hew to the science behind opioid addiction and related public policy. Their book will help people who use drugs and their families, health professionals, and policy makers make wiser and safer choices for themselves and their communities"
—**Hilary Kunins, Assistant Commissioner,**
Bureau of Alcohol and Drug Use,
New York City Department of Health and Mental Hygiene

"This highly informative book is a valuable resource to help families truly understand addiction. Most, if not all, of your questions will be answered."
—**Toni Torsch, Director, Daniel Carl Torsch Foundation**

"*The Opioid Epidemic* offers insightful life-saving educational information not only for health professionals but for the millions of individuals and families struggling to find answers in a sea of confusion and conflicting information. An important contribution from two of the most informed and practiced thought-leaders on solving the opioid crisis."
—**Greg Williams, Executive Vice President, Facing Addiction**

THE OPIOID EPIDEMIC
WHAT EVERYONE NEEDS TO KNOW®

YNGVILD OLSEN
Institutes for Behavior Resources, Inc.

JOSHUA M. SHARFSTEIN
Johns Hopkins Bloomberg School of Public Health

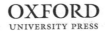
OXFORD
UNIVERSITY PRESS

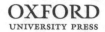

OXFORD
UNIVERSITY PRESS

Oxford University Press is a department of the University of Oxford. It furthers
the University's objective of excellence in research, scholarship, and education
by publishing worldwide. Oxford is a registered trade mark of Oxford University
Press in the UK and certain other countries.

"What Everyone Needs to Know" is a registered trademark of
Oxford University Press.

Published in the United States of America by Oxford University Press
198 Madison Avenue, New York, NY 10016, United States of America.

© Oxford University Press 2019

CIP data is on file at the Library of Congress
ISBN 978-0-19-091602-2 (pbk.)
ISBN 978-0-19-091603-9 (hbk.)

This material is not intended to be, and should not be considered, a substitute
for medical or other professional advice. Treatment for the conditions described
in this material is highly dependent on the individual circumstances. And,
while this material is designed to offer accurate information with respect to the
subject matter covered and to be current as of the time it was written, research
and knowledge about medical and health issues is constantly evolving and
dose schedules for medications are being revised continually, with new side
effects recognized and accounted for regularly. Readers must therefore always
check the product information and clinical procedures with the most up-to-date
published product information and data sheets provided by the manufacturers
and the most recent codes of conduct and safety regulation. The publisher and the
authors make no representations or warranties to readers, express or implied, as
to the accuracy or completeness of this material. Without limiting the foregoing,
the publisher and the authors make no representations or warranties as to the
accuracy or efficacy of the drug dosages mentioned in the material. The authors
and the publisher do not accept, and expressly disclaim, any responsibility for
any liability, loss or risk that may be claimed or incurred as a consequence of the
use and/or application of any of the contents of this material.

1 3 5 7 9 8 6 4 2

Paperback printed by Sheridan Books, Inc., United States of America
Hardback printed by Bridgeport National Bindery, Inc., United States of America

To Our Parents

CONTENTS

Section 2: Individuals and Families

2 Use of Opioid Medications for Pain   29

3 Misuse of Opioids   43

4 Opioid Addiction   51

5 Opioid Overdose   61

6 Treatment for Opioid Addiction 67

14 Harm Reduction Policy for the Opioid Epidemic 191

15 Criminal Justice Policy and the Opioid Epidemic 205

PREFACE

The taps on the shoulder are discreet, the words whispered in shame. "My son is in jail again." "I worry every day that my daughter might die." "Why is my husband behaving like this?" "My wife overdosed last night." "I think I might have a problem."

For a crisis that has landed on millions of doorsteps across the country, the opioid epidemic has left many individuals and families in a state of isolation—as well as in a state of confusion. Confusion about what opioids are. About how addiction develops. About which treatments work. About how best to support the process of recovery. Out of desperation, many Americans have spent their savings on worthless programs and false cures.

Misunderstanding about opioids also pervades community meeting rooms, town councils, city and state agencies, and the halls of power in Washington, D.C. It permeates emergency departments, physician offices, and hospital wards. More than 70,000 Americans each year are dying of overdose, the majority from opioids. The crisis is responsible for a decline in life expectancy in America over the past three years. Yet many responses are constructed with little awareness of evidence or history. The result is that many of the actions taken to address the opioid epidemic have made little difference—or even made the problem worse.

This state of confusion on opioids is, in its own way, a national crisis.

In our own careers, the two of us spend many hours answering questions about opioids from individuals with addiction, friends and family members, clinicians, agency officials, and elected leaders. Some of these conversations happen in person during work hours; others in urgent calls late at night.

One of us is a doctor specializing in addiction medicine; the other is a former public health official. We have witnessed the devastating consequences of the opioid epidemic. But we have also seen many people heal and recover.

We share this conviction: The fog that surrounds the opioid epidemic is not impenetrable.

With effective treatment, people can feel better, reunite with their families, and regain faith in themselves. With greater understanding, families can become an essential source of support to their loved ones. With an informed perspective, communities can tackle the opioid crisis as a solvable problem. With a public health approach, measuring results at each step, our nation can turn the corner on the opioid epidemic.

Our purpose in writing this book is to document the lessons of science and history, to replace myths with facts, and to help individuals, families, and policymakers tell the difference between wishful thinking and what really works. Of course, there is much unknown about opioid addiction. But what is known can be put to great use.

It starts with the basics: What are opioids, and how do they affect the human brain and body. The book's first section explains the essential concepts of tolerance, withdrawal, and physical dependence—and how these differ from addiction. This section discusses effective treatment and recovery and ends with an overview of the opioid epidemic and what can be done.

Individuals and families need straightforward answers. The book's second section addresses when to use opioids for pain and why opioids are misused. It answers questions on addiction and treatment, including for teenagers and pregnant women. It covers how to stop an overdose in progress and how to assist a loved one in recovery.

Why did the opioid epidemic start, and how can it be stopped? The third section addresses urgent questions facing local communities, cities and counties, and states,—as well as the federal government. This section reviews the evidence on which programs and policies work for prevention and treatment—and which do not. It also addresses sensitive issues, including the "not in my backyard" syndrome, the "war on drugs," and the evidence about harm reduction approaches such as naloxone distribution, syringe services programs, and overdose prevention sites (also known as supervised consumption spaces). It closes with specific recommendations to save lives.

At times, it may seem that opioids leave us all powerless to resist their devastation. But this is not true. "Knowledge is power," wrote philosopher Francis Bacon more than 400 years ago. With greater understanding can come strength, resolve, and hope.

ACKNOWLEDGMENTS

This is a book two careers in the making. We thank everyone who made these careers possible, from our earliest mentors to our many amazing colleagues at IBR/REACH, the Maryland Department of Health, Behavioral Health System Baltimore, the American Society of Addiction Medicine, and the Johns Hopkins Bloomberg School of Public Health.

Individuals with opioid addiction, along with their friends and family members, have been our greatest teachers. We are profoundly grateful to have shared in their journeys. We also deeply appreciate the community leaders and policymakers who have trusted us amid crisis.

We appreciate the tireless efforts of our research assistant Jenny Wen and the helpful comments of Kathleen Rebbert-Franklin, Sarah Despres, Sean Allen, and Colleen Barry. This book would not have been possible without the able assistance of Chloe Layman and the expert guidance and generous encouragement of our editor Chad Zimmerman, both at Oxford University Press.

Finally, we thank Sam and Isak, two remarkable young men who keep us hopeful for the future (and grounded in the present). In writing this book, we are honoring the tradition of our parents, Marie, Bjorn, Margaret, and Steven. All four are physicians devoted to improving the lives of others through science, care, and compassion. This book is for them.

Section 1

THE BASICS

1

THE BASICS OF OPIOIDS AND OPIOID ADDICTION

What are opioids?

Opioids are a group of chemical compounds that can reduce pain, cause sensations of pleasure, and induce sleep. To have these and other effects on the human body, all opioids interact with specific receptors on the surface of cells called opioid receptors.

How are opioids made?

There are four sources of opioids.

Agriculture

The oldest known opioids come directly from the seeds of the poppy plant, *Papaver Somniferum*. The history of the poppy plant stretches back more than 5,000 years to a time when ancient Sumerians, the earliest known civilization in today's Iraq, discovered the "Hul Gil" or "joy plant."[1]

Today, poppy plants are grown for the pharmaceutical production of opioids under the supervision of the United Nations in Australia, France, Hungary, India, Spain, and Turkey.[2] Poppies are also grown illicitly in Afghanistan, Mexico, and other warm and dry areas of Central Asia and Latin America.

Cutting open poppy seeds yields opium, a milky fluid that can be hardened into a resin. Pharmaceutical companies extract morphine, codeine, and thebaine from this resin. Opium can also be cooked and then smoked, eaten, or injected.[3] All opioids that come directly from the poppy plant are known as *opiates*.

Agriculture plus the laboratory

At the turn of the 20th century, the German company Bayer Pharmaceuticals began to modify opiates to create new types of opioids. In 1898, Bayer announced its first product: a derivative of morphine to treat cough, to be marketed under the brand name of "heroin." (This invention did not proceed as planned.)

The opiate thebaine is the source of several other "semisynthetic" opioids used widely in medicine today, including oxycodone and hydrocodone, used for pain, as well as buprenorphine, which is used for pain as well as to treat opioid addiction.

The laboratory alone

The last 50 years has seen the emergence of a third group of opioids: those made entirely in the laboratory, with no involvement of the poppy plant. The "synthetic" opioids include methadone, an opioid used mainly to treat opioid addiction but which can also be used for pain and fentanyl, a particularly strong opioid used in hospitals for anesthesia and to treat severe cancer pain.

Outside of the pharmaceutical industry, unauthorized laboratories produce varieties of opioids. Since 2013, these laboratories have been producing fentanyl and a series of closely related chemical compounds. These synthetic opioids are responsible for an increasing number of overdose deaths.

The human body

There is one final source of opioids: the human body. The body's own opioids affect the experience of pain, pleasure, and reward. When websites advise 10 ways to "boost your endorphins," they're trying to stimulate your body to make more opioids.

How do opioids affect the brain?

Opioids can change perceptions of pain and pleasure, alter levels of alertness and breathing, and impact memory. These and other effects are the result of opioids binding to specific opioid receptors on nerve cells in different parts of the brain, much like different keys fitting into different locks. Each combination of lock and key results in a specific effect on the nerve cell and, therefore, a specific effect on the brain.

Pain

Opioids reduce the sensation of pain. When opioids bind to certain opioid receptors in the brain and spinal cord, changes in the nerve cells alter how pain signals are transmitted and processed. The result is a dulling of the pain, even with an injury still present.

Alertness and breathing

Many opioids reduce alertness and slow breathing through their effect on specific opioid receptors in the brainstem. This can be a useful effect. In the operating room, anesthesiologists routinely administer certain opioids to put their patients to sleep, with machines on hand to control breathing. However, outside of such a controlled environment, high doses of opioids can cause people to fall deeply asleep and then stop breathing entirely.

Pleasure

Opioids can affect the perception of pleasure through the brain's "reward pathway." This pathway involves a set of nerve cells deep in the brain that, when their opioid receptors are activated, release the chemical dopamine. This release of dopamine is then responsible for generating the sensations of pleasure and reward. For example, endorphins, the body's own opioids, trigger the release of dopamine from these cells naturally—such as after a great meal, during an exhilarating run, and at the moment of an orgasm. (This last effect is why biologists credit the brain's "reward pathway" for the survival of the human race.)

Pharmaceutical and illicit opioids can also bind to the same specific receptors and activate these cells; in some people, under the right circumstances, the result can be the release of large quantities of dopamine, causing an intense perception of pleasure and commandeering the brain's reward system.

Memory

At the same time that an opioid is binding to one receptor and triggering a large release of dopamine to cause an intense feeling of pleasure, it may bind to another type of receptor on the surface of special cells involved in memory. It may be partly through this process that the brain learns what external triggers, or cues, are associated with a feeling of pleasure or reward. This association may be one reason why people who return to the place where they once misused opioids, even years later, can feel an intense craving again.

Here's a case example: A 45-year old man with an opioid addiction leaves prison after serving a 6-year sentence for armed robbery. He had used heroin for over 10 years before his arrest, but he did not use once while incarcerated. The bus taking him home passes the corner where he regularly bought heroin. All of a sudden, he feels butterflies in his stomach, his hands and forehead break out in a sweat, and he senses an intense warmth surge through his body. As his mind hungers and aches, he tries to shove the craving aside. The bus turns the corner, but he has already jumped off. He begins another 3 years of destructive heroin use—during which time he overdoses twice and becomes infected with HIV—before seeking treatment.

How do opioids affect the body?

Opioid receptors are found not only on cells in the brain and spinal cord but also in the skin, eyes, nasal passages, lungs, bones, and the gastrointestinal tract. The administration of opioids, therefore, can affect many parts of the body—typically in a manner that could be characterized as slowing or inhibiting. Opioids can cause constipation, dry eyes, dry mouth, lowered sex drive, and difficulty urinating.

What forms do opioids take?

Opioids take multiple forms. For example, morphine is manufactured for oral, injection, or rectal delivery. Fentanyl can be made into a skin patch, a liquid spray for use in the nose or under the tongue, a solution for intravenous use, and a powder that can be compressed into tablets or flattened into a film that is placed under the tongue or pressed against the inside of the cheek.

The way an opioid reaches the brain matters. The faster an opioid gets to the brain, the greater the chance it will lead to addiction. An opioid in a form that is injected or sprayed in the nose enters the bloodstream and reaches the brain within seconds. An opioid that is inhaled moves from the lungs to the bloodstream and to the brain quickly as well. By contrast, when taken by mouth, an opioid passes through the esophagus and the stomach and then into the intestines before it is absorbed into the bloodstream. The bloodstream then carries the opioid through the liver before it reaches the brain. This typically ends minutes to hours later with only a fraction of the opioid initially taken by mouth actually reaching the brain. A delayed process also takes place with opioids absorbed through skin patches.

This biology explains why people who misuse opioids typically melt or crush up tablets and powders to either inject, snort, or inhale. It is also why a person with opioid addiction will extract fentanyl from a skin patch and inject it rather than wear the patch on their arm for an effect.

How do opioids differ from one another?

Opioids differ from each other in several important ways.

First, some opioids are more potent than others. *Potency* refers to how much of the opioid is needed to achieve a certain effect. For example, only a couple of milligrams of the opioid hydromorphone produces pain relief in most people. But it generally takes 30 milligrams of the less potent opioid codeine to produce the same pain relief as just a couple milligrams of hydromorphone. As this example illustrates, opioids cannot be compared milligram to milligram when predicting or describing their effects.

Certain opioids, such as fentanyl, are so potent that their doses are measured in micrograms, which are 1000 times smaller than milligrams. This means a miniscule amount of fentanyl produces the same effects as a couple milligrams of hydromorphone or 30 milligrams of codeine. Fentanyl's high potency is one reason it is so dangerous when illicitly produced and sold on the street.

There are reference tables that help compare the potency of various opioids, but these are just general guides for predicting effects on individual patients. That's because people differ in how their bodies respond to different opioids. One person, for example, might experience a lot of pain relief from a single dose of codeine, while another person only notices nausea and vomiting from the same medication at the same dose.

Second, some opioids last longer in the human body than others. For example, codeine lasts only a few hours in the body. As a result, people who receive this medication for pain often take several doses a day. By contrast, one dose of methadone per day to treat opioid addiction is enough to maintain a steady level in the bloodstream. That's why treatment programs provide for once-a-day dosing of methadone, like primary care doctors prescribing a once-a-day dose of a blood pressure medicine.

Third, some opioids move into the brain faster than others. This quality has to do with how easily the opioid dissolves in fat, a characteristic necessary to pass through the barrier that separates the bloodstream from the brain's nerve cells. Opioids that are very "fat soluble" include heroin and fentanyl—two substances that, not coincidentally, are highly prone to misuse and addiction.

Fourth, opioids differ in their effects on opioid receptors. One opioid's stimulation of a receptor may lead to the full activation of the nerve cell, while another opioid's effect on the same receptor may result only in a partial activation of the cell. This subtle difference explains why the opioid buprenorphine has less of an effect on breathing than most other opioids.

Fifth, opioids differ in how avidly they bind to receptors. This means that if two opioids are taken together, one will outcompete the other for space on the receptor and, therefore, for effects on the brain. Up to a certain point, the medication methadone can outcompete heroin, which explains why treatment with methadone offers a degree of protection from overdose, even in case of relapse.

What is tolerance to opioids?

The body adapts to opioids after just a few days, so that increasing amounts may be needed to have the same effects. This process, known as *tolerance*, develops because the opioid receptors on the surface of cells become desensitized to the opioids and because cells start to produce fewer opioid receptors.

The good news

Tolerance develops to the sedating effects of opioids, making it less likely that people with pain will feel tired after taking their opioid medications. In addition, as individuals develop tolerance to the respiratory effects of opioids, the risk for overdose declines.

The bad news

People also may develop tolerance to the pain-relieving effects of opioids. When this happens, they may need a higher dose to get the same relief. Unfortunately, the higher dose brings along a greater degree of sedation and an increased risk of overdose.

People who experience pleasure with opioids also learn quickly that tolerance develops to this effect too. This means that people who are addicted to opioids find themselves seeking out higher doses and more potent opioids, often in an unsuccessful attempt to experience the same degree of pleasure associated with the first time they used an opioid.

Tolerance does not develop to all opioid effects. For example, tolerance does not develop to constipation from opioids. As a result, people who use opioids and develop constipation should not expect this unpleasant condition to go away with time.

Loss of tolerance

When people are no longer exposed to opioids, their bodies revert over a period of days to their original state. This means that just a small dose of opioids, again, will have a significant effect—and it also means that if the dose is too high, it may have a lethal effect. The loss of tolerance can be very dangerous.

Here's a case example: A young woman who has snorted prescription oxycodone for a year has developed tolerance to its effects on breathing. She is arrested for stealing pills from her neighbor's house. In jail, without access to opioids, she loses tolerance over a period of days. Once released, she has cravings to use again. She buys oxycodone pills from a friend, snorting her usual dose. Having lost tolerance, she overdoses.

This biology explains why people with opioid addiction face an elevated risk of death after release from detention, especially in the absence of effective treatment.[4]

What is opioid withdrawal?

Opioid withdrawal is a series of symptoms experienced by people who have been taking at least 60 milligrams of morphine or its equivalent for more than a week or so and then quickly cut back or abruptly stop. Withdrawal occurs because the brain, skin, eyes, nose, bones, and intestinal tract, which became used to the presence of opioids, now respond to their absence.

The symptoms of withdrawal can be thought of as the opposite of the effects of taking opioids. Common symptoms include feelings of restlessness and agitation, chills, sweats, runny eyes and nose, yawning, muscle and joint aches, abdominal cramps, diarrhea, nausea, and vomiting. Since opioid responses vary by person, the experience of withdrawal varies, too.

Opioid withdrawal occurs in two main phases: an initial phase and a protracted phase. The initial phase is the most severe. Many compare the experience to suffering from a bad case of flu—or to being run over by a truck. While opioid withdrawal is not typically fatal, some have died from severe dehydration associated with nausea, vomiting, and diarrhea.[5]

The onset, severity, and duration of withdrawal symptoms in any individual depends on the type of opioid used, as well as the dose, the method of use, and the length of time of use. For example, someone who has injected heroin multiple times a day for many years will experience more rapid onset of more severe withdrawal symptoms, but for a shorter period of time, than someone who has taken the relatively low dose of 10 mg of methadone daily for a year.

"Protracted opioid withdrawal" is the name given to the restlessness, irritability, insomnia, and general fatigue that people often report even after the initial phase symptoms have disappeared. Some studies have also found persistent abnormalities in vital signs such as blood pressure and respiratory rate.[6] Lasting as long as a year after the last use of opioids, this period is an especially vulnerable time for relapse.

What is physical dependence on opioids?

Physical dependence is a concept closely tied to tolerance and withdrawal. Someone might (accurately) say, "My body has become tolerant to opioids, and if I stopped using abruptly, I would experience withdrawal. That means I am now physically dependent."

Opioids are far from the only substances that have these kinds of effects on the human body. People develop physical dependence marked by tolerance and withdrawal to alcohol, nicotine, caffeine, and certain medications, including benzodiazepines (such as Xanax®), some antidepressants, and certain anti-hypertensive medications.

A key point: The development of physical dependence is a function of biology alone. It does not include counterproductive behaviors. Someone taking oxycodone to treat pain caused by cancer will develop physical dependence, just like someone using heroin. Indeed, everyone who takes the equivalent of 60 mg of morphine a day for about a week will develop physical dependence.

Physical dependence and addiction are two different concepts. Unlike physical dependence, addiction involves counterproductive behaviors. Addiction is defined by craving, compulsive drug-seeking, and continued use despite negative consequences. It also reflects dysfunction in the brain circuits involved in reward, learning, memory, and motivation. Many people who take opioids regularly and appropriately for pain control or for addiction treatment become physically dependent on their treatment medications but do not develop an addiction to them.

What is opioid addiction?

Addiction is characterized by pathological craving and compulsion that drives someone to keep using a substance even in the face of severe negative consequences to the person's life, including the threat of death. (Formal definitions of addiction are included in Appendix 1.) Along with many other legal and illegal drugs, opioids can cause addiction.

Here's a case example: A middle-aged man starts taking opioids as prescribed after a knee injury. He continues taking them after the pain is gone because he likes the pleasurable feeling the medication gives him. Running out of medicine, he begins to "borrow" doses from friends or neighbors. He also learns that he can get a more intense pleasurable feeling if he crushes up the tablets and snorts them. He goes from doctor to doctor making up new symptoms in search of opioid prescriptions, because he feels he cannot function without them. His brain remembers that wonderful pleasurable feeling from his first time snorting pills. Even when he is fired from his job and confronted with the prospect of losing his family, he is not able to stop his use.

Here's another case example: A young woman prescribed oxycodone for a leg injury requires higher and higher doses for pain relief. She starts misusing the pills, leading her doctor to stop prescribing them. She turns to illicit heroin on the street.

Over the next several years, she injects heroin until wounds in her legs are so severe that she cannot walk. She pays someone to carry her up the stairs of an abandoned building to buy heroin and to help her to inject it. Later, the young woman tells her doctor, "When I started taking extra oxys for my leg, I swore that I would never use heroin, much less inject it. I still don't understand how this all happened."

Underlying these behaviors is a brain disease. Scientists have found that addiction involves disruption of and functional changes in the circuits of the brain that regulate reward and pleasure, as well as motivation, impulse control, stress response, judgment, and self-awareness.[7]

Opioid addiction is a chronic illness. This means there is no cure and that there is always a risk of relapse. The goal, therefore, becomes lifelong management of the disease. Like other chronic diseases, opioid addiction is not static across a person's life. There are times when symptoms are present, and there are periods of remission, when the disease is stable.

Some people disagree with calling opioid addiction a chronic illness. They argue that because addiction involves counterproductive behavior, it cannot be a disease of the brain. This is a fallacy. Counterproductive behaviors are an integral part of many other chronic illnesses. For example, eating too much sugar, fat, and salt can lead to adult-onset diabetes or worsen high blood pressure. Many patients with these chronic conditions control their symptoms through diet and regular exercise.

A related term to opioid addiction is *opioid use disorder*. Opioid use disorder is the name for the condition that a clinician diagnoses in a person with opioid addiction.

What is the stigma of addiction?

Many people consider those with addiction to be moral failures, lacking sufficient will power, and consciously choosing to destroy their lives with alcohol or other drugs. These attitudes reflect a deep stigma that goes back more than 100 years in the United States.

In the early 20th century, when drug use became illegal across the United States and much of the world, people who used drugs became criminals—incarcerated rather than cared for. Even after scientific research clarified the understanding of addiction as a brain disease, punitive approaches and beliefs about addiction as a moral failing have persisted. Stigma has led to ongoing bias toward, and discrimination against, people who have an addiction.

For example, a public opinion survey published in 2014 found that 90% of American adults would not want someone with an addiction to marry into their family. This compares to 59% of adults asked the same for someone with mental illness.[8] According to the survey, most American adults support the ability of landlords to deny housing to people with addiction, 76% oppose public housing subsidies for those with addiction, and 78% would not want to work with someone with an addiction.

Bias and discrimination against those with addiction is reflected in the language used to talk about the disease and those affected by it. For example, words such as "junkie," "addict," and "abuse" all conjure up images of people with addiction as dirty, at fault, and unworthy. This is a false stereotype.

The most accurate language is clear and non-judgmental—the same language that is used for other chronic illnesses. This means, for example, placing the person first—not the disease. So instead of "heroin addict," one should say "a person with addiction to heroin." Instead of calling a person with an addiction "clean," the appropriate term is "in remission" or "in recovery." Instead of labeling a urine drug test "dirty," it is better to say "expected" or "unexpected" or "positive for [a particular substance] or negative for [a particular substance]."

Stigmatizing language does not assist the care of someone with addiction. For example, unless there is actual dirt in a urine specimen cup, labeling the drug test result as "dirty" does not help the physician or the patient in understanding a response to treatment or the status of an illness. The drug test is a laboratory test just like any other test performed in medicine; the results should be described using precise medical terms.

Using appropriate language matters. One study found that mental health professionals thought far more negatively about a "substance abuser" in a clinical scenario than about "a person with a substance use disorder" in an otherwise identical situation.[9]

In 2015, the White House Office of the National Drug Control Policy published a list of preferred terms to use related to addiction.[10] In 2017, the Associated Press released a glossary of non-stigmatizing terminology for journalists to use in covering the opioid epidemic.[11] Adopting non-judgmental terminology is an important, effective, low-cost step that can serve as a measure for broader changes in attitudes and perceptions toward people with addiction. Appendix 2 includes suggested language to use with respect to addiction.

Is there a cure for opioid addiction?

Unfortunately, no. Doctors, researchers, families, and people with addiction themselves have looked for a cure for opioid addiction for hundreds of years, often trying all sorts of remedies. Many people have died from these "cures."[12]

Today, the Internet offers an array of products and services promising quick fixes for opioid addiction. These include dietary supplements with names like "CalmSupport" and "Opiate Freedom 5-Pack,"[13] luxurious "rehab clinics," an untested hallucinogen called ibogaine, a botanical called kratom, and even marijuana. Distraught families can be vulnerable to misinformation and deception. Many have spent thousands of dollars in a desperate, and often dangerous, search for a miracle cure.

Can the symptoms of opioid addiction improve without treatment?

In some cases, yes. A certain percentage of people who misuse opioids or even use heroin are able to stop without treatment, never to use again. This was the case with a large number of soldiers who used opium and heroin while in Vietnam during the Vietnam war, but who, upon returning to the United States, did not continue to do so.[14]

Spontaneous recovery in opioid addiction is not well understood—just as it is often not well understood for other conditions, such as diabetes and even cancer. It may be that those individuals who stop on their own and never use again do not have all of the characteristic brain changes of addiction. The fact that some people may achieve a spontaneous recovery does not mean that forgoing treatment is a recommended approach. Many people who try to stop on their own fail, and some die of an overdose in the process.

Is there effective treatment for opioid addiction?

Absolutely, yes. For the past 50 years, significant progress has been made in the treatment of opioid addiction. With effective, proven care, millions of people with opioid addiction now manage their disease and lead productive, meaningful lives.

Effective treatment has several components: medication, counseling and other clinical services, and social support. Two effective medications for opioid addiction are opioids themselves: buprenorphine and methadone. At therapeutic doses, these medications address some of the biochemical changes that cause the symptoms of addiction, without causing a sensation of pleasure. Their use often results in far less craving for illicit opioids and an end to counterproductive behaviors.

Patients turn their attention from seeking their next dose of illicit opioids to, for example, making amends with friends and family. One person suffering from an opioid addiction explained that she felt "married to heroin," and it was methadone that granted her a divorce.

A third medication more recently approved for opioid addiction, naltrexone, blocks the effects of opioids in the brain. It can be taken in daily pills or in a monthly injection, known as depot naltrexone.

In addition to medication, treatment for opioid addiction often includes counseling, which can be delivered in a variety of settings. These locations range from community-based programs and primary care offices to residential treatment centers. Most people with opioid addiction do well receiving care on an outpatient basis near where they live. All people with addiction need social support, including healthy friendships and access to nutritious food, safe housing, and, for many people, employment.

Treatment for opioid addiction is as or more effective than treatment for many other chronic illnesses, including heart disease, diabetes, and cancer. Many studies have found success for as many as 75% of patients who receive effective treatment.[15,16,17,18,19,20,21] And there is ongoing research both to find better ways of providing existing treatments and to develop new therapies altogether.

Is taking methadone or buprenorphine just "replacing one addiction for another"?

No. People who take the opioids methadone and buprenorphine appropriately to treat opioid addiction are not addicted to these medications. Addiction is defined by craving, compulsive drug-seeking, and continued use despite negative consequences. Individuals in successful treatment and recovery no longer experience these symptoms.

Unfortunately, many people—including some who work in the addiction field—hold the mistaken view that taking methadone or buprenorphine is "replacing one addiction for another." For this reason, many residential treatment programs refuse to allow their patients to take the medications, and many 12-step programs do not permit people who do to hold leadership positions or even to speak at meetings.

Discrimination against people taking medications for addiction treatment is also common in other areas of society. Patients have been fired from their jobs after their employer found out they took methadone. Pregnant women have been told to stop taking their medication immediately after delivery or lose custody of their newborn child. The healthcare profession is not immune to this bias. Some pharmacists have refused to fill prescriptions for buprenorphine because they "don't believe" in the treatment.[22]

In the fall of 2017, Food and Drug Administration (FDA) Commissioner Scott Gottlieb testified before Congress about the use of medications for addiction treatment. He started by saying,

> Addiction requires the continued use of opioids despite harmful consequences. Addiction involves a psychological craving above and beyond a physical dependence. Someone who neglects his family, has trouble holding a job, or commits crimes to obtain opioids has an addiction. But someone who is physically dependent on opioids as a result of the treatment of pain but who is not craving more or harming themselves or others is not addicted.

He continued: "The same principle applies to medications used to treat opioid addiction. Someone who requires long-term treatment for opioid addiction with medications—including those that cause a physical dependence—is not addicted to those medications." He concluded, "We should not consider people who hold jobs, re-engage with their families, and regain control over their lives through treatment that uses medications to be addicted. Rather, we should consider them to be role models in the fight against the opioid epidemic."[23]

How do opioids cause overdose?

Opioids cause overdose by suppressing breathing. Typically, an adult at rest needs to take between 12 and 16 breaths per minute to maintain adequate levels of oxygen; fewer than 6 breaths per minute may be life-threatening. After about 5 minutes without sufficient oxygen, the heart slows and brain cells begin to die. This is also the point at which the levels of carbon dioxide and other toxins produced by the body start to poison other organs. Within minutes, this damage becomes irreversible, leading to death.

What is naloxone?

Naloxone is a medication that rapidly reverses opioid overdoses and saves lives. Once paramedics, police officers, and other bystanders arrive at the scene of an overdose, they aim to deliver naloxone as quickly as possible. One option is to inject the medication into a muscle, often with the needle going right through the patient's clothes. Another option is to squeeze the medication out of an inhaler directly into the person's nose.

Whether injected or inhaled, naloxone travels right to the brain and blocks the binding of opioids to receptors. Naloxone outcompetes opioids for the receptors, effectively reversing their effects. The result is that within seconds to minutes, the person starts breathing again and wakes up.

Mission accomplished? Not so fast.

Some people may wake up and leave the scene, only to die of an overdose several hours later—even without taking any more opioids.

The reason for delayed overdose is that naloxone begins to dissipate as soon as it is given. After several hours, the levels of naloxone have fallen considerably. If the opioid that caused the overdose persists longer in the body than the naloxone—as many opioids do—there is a risk for another overdose. This is why it is critical for people to seek medical attention following the reversal of an overdose, even if they seem to have recovered completely.

What are remission and recovery?

Remission is a state of substantial improvement in the symptoms of addiction. Remission means no longer misusing opioids and putting the pieces of a normal life back together. *Recovery* is a process of continual growth as people with addiction manage their disease to live productive, fulfilling, and meaningful lives. Several commonly used definitions of recovery are provided in Appendix 3.

A common misconception about opioid addiction is that recovery is rare—that most people spiral downward until they lose all their money, their families, their health, and, ultimately, their lives. Fueling this misconception is the fact that some people with severe addiction are highly visible, suffering in the light of day at street corners asking for money. Yet, there are many more people in recovery, often passing through the same street corners, either in cars or on foot. But it's impossible to spot them, because they look like everyone else.

What is relapse?

Relapse refers to a return to misusing prescription or illicit opioids after having achieved remission and recovery from opioid addiction. Some people in the addiction field distinguish "relapse" from a "lapse." They note that a lapse may be a one-time or a short-lived period of use without the recurrence of the negative consequences associated with the addiction.

Relapse, on the other hand, includes a return to continuous use accompanied by the problems that brings.

A critical question to ask after a lapse or a relapse is, "Why?" The answer may be that the person stopped taking their treatment medication. Or it may be that the person experienced a trigger that had not been previously recognized. Many people who relapse re-engage in treatment, and, with greater awareness of their vulnerabilities, achieve a more stable recovery. The National Institutes of Health advises that rather than give up, "the person [who has relapsed] needs to speak with their doctor to resume treatment, modify it, or try another treatment."[24]

Recently, some addiction medicine physicians have called for dropping the term "relapse" in favor of "recurrence," a more neutral medical term.[25]

What is the opioid epidemic?

The opioid epidemic refers to the enormous surge in opioid addiction and overdose over the last several decades in the United States. Much of the epidemic has its origins in medical practice. Starting in the 1990s, physicians in the United States began prescribing opioids for pain at rates three to four times higher than elsewhere in the world. A percentage of their patients developed an opioid addiction as a result. Then, the nation's cities, suburbs, and rural areas experienced major increases in heroin use. A recent surge of illicit fentanyl has driven the number of deaths from overdose to unprecedented levels.

There have been many attempts to make real the vast scale of the suffering caused by the opioid epidemic. One approach is to tell the stories of the epidemic's victims. In December 2016, *STAT* compiled the obituaries of people who died from overdose across the country in a feature titled "52 Weeks, 52 Faces."[26] In September 2017, the *Cincinnati Enquirer* published "Seven Days of Heroin: This Is What an Epidemic Looks

Like," a Pulitzer Prize–winning account of the experiences of individuals and families in Cincinnati.[27] And, in February 2018, *TIME* published an explicit series of photos and videos entitled "The Opioid Diaries."[28]

Others cite data. According to the most recent national survey, an estimated 2.2 million Americans suffer from addiction to opioids over the course of a year.[29] There is a zone of suffering and trauma around every individual with opioid addiction. Millions have been incarcerated, with criminal records limiting their opportunities to support their families. A growing number of children are experiencing abuse and neglect.[30] Employers report that the opioid crisis is undermining the labor force by reducing the pool of eligible workers.[31] Communities with overwhelmed social services, police departments, and ambulance services struggle to invest in education and economic development.

From a financial perspective, healthcare costs associated with the opioid epidemic are estimated at over $25 billion a year, and criminal justice costs in excess of $5 billion. The cost of lost productivity is even greater. In November 2017, the US Council of Economic Advisers estimated that the crisis is costing the US economy $504 billion dollars every year.[32]

The most visible consequences of the epidemic relate to health. Hundreds of thousands of people are arriving at emergency departments after overdosing each year. Intravenous drug use leads to HIV and hepatitis C infections, disfiguring skin abscesses, and life-threatening heart valve infections.[33] People with opioid addiction often neglect other chronic illnesses, including diabetes and depression, and often wind up dying from these other conditions decades earlier than they otherwise would.

Death by overdose is the final consequence of the opioid epidemic. From fewer than 10,000 in 2001, overdose deaths related to opioids climbed past 47,000 in 2017—more than from traffic fatalities, from guns, from AIDS at the peak of the HIV epidemic, and from combat at the peak of the Vietnam War. White

Americans are about twice as likely as African Americans to have an opioid addiction, but as a result of the recent surge in fentanyl, the rate of death among African Americans is rising more quickly.[34]

Opioid-related deaths now represent about 1.5% of all US fatalities, including 20% of deaths among adults between 24 and 35 years of age.[35] Some experts expect more than 500,000 additional deaths in the next decade.[36]

With so many overdose victims in their 20s, 30s, 40s, and 50s, the opioid epidemic is reducing US life expectancy. After years of increase, US life expectancy began to plateau in 2010 and then actually decline in 2015, the first decrease since AIDS in the early 1990s. In 2017, life expectancy dropped again, the first three-year decline since World War I and the Great Influenza, a century ago.[37]

What can be done to respond effectively to the opioid epidemic?

For the last century, the primary response of the United States to opioid addiction has been prohibition and criminalization. There have also been periodic investments in research, treatment, and other services. To save the most lives in the shortest amount of time, the nation should fully embrace a public health approach to this challenge.

A public health approach includes three basic steps: assessment, policy development, and assurance.[38] Assessment means using the best available data to understand the problem and potential solutions. Without access to timely information, it is too easy to rely on assumptions and misunderstandings about what is happening or what is to be done. Unfortunately, most places in the United States still lack access to specific, usable data on opioids.

Policy development means using research and evidence—not assumptions or ideology—to design a strategy. There are some great examples of localities and states making the reversal medication naloxone, outreach services, and effective treatment programs more available – and these areas are starting to see results.[39] Yet far more common are policy agendas driven by moral judgment and fear, filled with approaches to treatment and law enforcement that are unsupported by data.

Assurance means constantly checking to be sure that programs and policies are having the intended impact, with adjustments at every step. Only by rigorously assessing what works can policies improve over time. Patience, however, is not a great American virtue.

Public health approaches are rarely flashy. Progress can be halting. Slowly but surely, the tools of public health chip away at problems until they are prevented, managed, or controlled. That's how public health strategies have succeeded in dramatically reducing the number of deaths from smoking, motor vehicle accidents, and infectious disease.

Sometimes promising approaches are controversial. It can be difficult for leaders to embrace politically unpopular ideas, even those that are likely to be successful. In this sense, the greatest challenge of the opioid epidemic may not be the opioids themselves. It may be the difficult fact that what is the right thing to do may feel to many like exactly the wrong thing to do. And that what feels like the right thing to do might make matters worse.

Here's the bottom line: Not all well-intentioned approaches to addressing the opioid epidemic are good ideas. Some are based on evidence and experience; others, on misunderstanding, blame, fear, or frustration. What's needed for success is the wisdom—and the courage—to tell the difference.[40]

Section 2

INDIVIDUALS AND FAMILIES

2

USE OF OPIOID MEDICATIONS FOR PAIN

When is it appropriate for someone to receive opioids for pain?

Sometimes. Taking opioids for pain might be necessary, or it might not be worth the risks. A few factors can help tell the difference. These include the following.

The severity of pain

Opioids should be reserved for severe pain. Many people with mild and even moderate pain respond well to approaches that do not involve medications, including physical therapy, acupuncture, and the passage of time. When medications are needed, nonopioid pain medications, including ibuprofen, often are sufficient. For example, most people who have their wisdom teeth extracted can manage their pain with ibuprofen (Motrin or Advil) and acetaminophen (Tylenol)—even though dentists and oral surgeons often prescribe days to weeks of opioid therapy.[1]

The type of pain

Patients who have severe pain from serious injuries or following major surgeries typically benefit from a short course of opioids. Opioids are also often necessary to treat the severe pain associated with cancer. However, patients with significant pain caused by nerve impingement or damage, called neuropathic pain, respond less well to opioids. These patients may get relief from other types of medications, including some originally developed for seizure disorders.

The duration of pain

There is ample evidence that opioids are effective for short-term, severe pain. However, there is little evidence for the effectiveness of long-term opioid therapy for chronic pain, typically defined as pain that lasts for 3 months or longer. While some individual patients may benefit from long-term opioid treatment, the risks often outweigh the benefits.

Special circumstances

Opioids are often helpful for palliative and end-of-life care.

Should opioids be used for chronic, non-cancer pain?

Rarely. Chronic pain—defined as pain for more than 3 months—often reflects a nervous system gone awry. It is normal to feel pain for days or weeks after an injury or surgery; this short-term sensation reflects tissue damage and the healing process. By comparison, chronic pain serves no biological or functional purpose.

A substantial minority of people with pain from an injury or surgery will go on to develop chronic pain. For these people, the injury has passed, but the nervous system has not reset. In these instances, the nervous system itself becomes a large part of the source of the pain. Chronic pain is now considered a disease onto itself because of its underlying mechanisms and because of its significant impacts on a person's life and function.

For some patients suffering from chronic pain, opioids may actually make the situation worse rather than better.[2] Opioids may be of limited benefit, while side effects continue to mount.

Patients living with chronic pain typically never become completely pain-free. So the goal of chronic pain management should be to focus on improving and sustaining function despite some pain. Effective regimens often include close monitoring of function, short trials of different therapies to find what works, and frequent assessments. A recent study of patients with chronic knee and back pain found that a combination of non-opioid pain medications and physical therapy was as effective in improving function and actually better at reducing pain as a regimen of opioid medications.[3]

In some instances, opioids are appropriate for patients with chronic pain—but only when there are specific, realistic goals in mind and when the patient and doctor are prepared to stop the medication if the goals are not met. Before and during opioid therapy for chronic pain, weighing the benefits and side effects on a regular basis is a critical step that can help avoid overdose and the development of addiction.

In what forms are opioid medications used for pain?

Eighteen different types of opioids are available in the United States for the treatment of pain.[4] These medications are sold in a multitude of forms under dozens of different product names, some of which are listed in Appendix 4.

Some opioids are combined with other medications in the same pill. For example, Percocet® pills include 5, 7.5, or 10 milligrams of the opioid oxycodone combined with 325 milligrams of acetaminophen, which is the active ingredient in Tylenol. The purpose of the combination is to use two different kinds of medications to achieve greater pain relief than either alone.

There's a hidden danger in these combination products, however. Unlike with opioids, tolerance does not develop to the effects of the companion drug. Those patients who, as a result of tolerance to opioids, increase their dose of combination products over time may suffer serious side effects. For example, patients who take too many Percocet® risk severe liver failure as a result of acetaminophen overdose.

Some opioids are available in "time release" preparations. These formulations are manufactured to release opioids far more slowly than usual, extending the time a single dose provides pain relief. To compensate for the less frequent administration, each pill contains a larger amount of the active ingredient. So, for example, instead of taking 20 milligrams of oxycodone four times a day, a patient can take 40 milligrams of time release oxycodone twice a day. (Time release oxycodone is marketed under the brand name OxyContin®.)

There are hidden dangers in time release preparations as well. One is that the time-release material of some preparations may easily and quickly degrade in the presence of alcohol, leading to a dumping of the entire opioid content of the capsule all at once—and risking overdose.

The second hidden danger is misuse. Because of the substantial amount of opioids in each pill, these medications are ripe targets for trouble. When people began to crush and inject OxyContin® tablets, for example, the nation's current opioid epidemic really began to pick up steam.

Should people with a family history of addiction worry about taking opioids for pain?

Yes. Addiction runs in families. About half of the risk of developing an addiction is based on genetics. Knowledge of a family history of addiction to marijuana, alcohol, cocaine, or opioids may help patients and their healthcare providers make better decisions about prescribing opioids for pain.

A patient with a significant history of addiction in his family may decline a few days of opioid therapy after a minor accident, even if the physician is ready to write a prescription to have opioids on hand, "just in case." When opioids are necessary for severe pain from a serious injury or major surgery, a patient and physician may decide to meet frequently to review how the treatment is progressing.

Here's a case example: A 25-year-old man with a strong family history of addiction develops a strong sensation of pleasure after a single dose of opioids given for an ankle injury. He recognizes that this is a warning sign that his brain may be especially sensitive to the rewarding effects of opioids. He tells his physician about the experience, and she switches him to a non-opioid pain medication immediately.

While research continues into the genetics of addiction, there is, unfortunately, no reliable genetic testing to help guide therapies such as opioids for pain.

What should I discuss with my doctor before taking opioids for pain?

Five good questions to ask your doctor before taking opioids for pain include:

- *Do I need to take opioids?* Many patients can manage mild to moderate pain with non-medication treatment, such as physical therapy or acupuncture, or non-opioid medications, such as ibuprofen.
- *For how long should I take the opioids?* For short-term pain, such as the pain from a minor surgery, most patients will need opioids for 3 days or less.
- *Will the opioids create a problem with any of my other medications?* For example, patients should avoid taking opioids for pain and a benzodiazepine such as diazepam (Valium®) or alprazolam (Xanax®) at the same time, because of the increased risk of overdose.[5]
- *What side effects should I watch out for?* Doctors should explain the risks of sedation as well as the warning signs of euphoria and craving that could increase the risk of misuse and addiction.
- *How will I know that the opioids are working?* This may be the most important question of all. Having a clear goal for treatment, especially for chronic pain, helps patients decide whether it makes sense to keep taking the

medications (and to keep being exposed to their risks)—
or taper off and try another approach.

Should I take an opioid medication if I am pregnant?

It depends. Every medication taken during pregnancy has the
potential to affect the developing fetus. Opioid medications
are no different. Most of the Food and Drug Administration–
approved opioid medications were designated as pregnancy
category C. This means: "Animal reproduction studies have
shown an adverse effect on the fetus and there are no adequate
and well-controlled studies in humans, but potential benefits
may warrant use of the drug in pregnant women despite potential risks."[6]

Not much help, is it? The high level of uncertainty means
that each situation has to be taken on its own. A pregnant
woman who suffers severe injuries in a car accident should
receive opioid medications for anesthesia in surgery and for
severe pain in recovery. The benefits to her far outweigh the
potential adverse effect on the fetus. At the same time, a pregnant woman who falls and sprains her ankle should try other
types of pain management before taking an opioid.

What are the side effects of opioid medications for pain?

Opioid side effects fall into two categories: the bothersome and
the serious.

All opioids share the same spectrum of side effects, but
not everyone who takes an opioid will experience all of these
symptoms or to the same degree.

Common bothersome side effects include:

• Constipation from the impact of opioids on the intestines.
Most patients taking opioids benefit from regular exercise, staying well hydrated with water, and a stool sof-
tener such as docusate to prevent constipation from

developing. Once constipation has developed, other measures, such as laxatives or enemas, may be needed in the short term, because stool softeners are minimally effective in treating this condition. In rare cases, constipation can turn into impaction, which is as bad as it sounds, and may even require hospitalization.
- Itching, which can be treated with ondansetron, an anti-nausea medicine.
- Nausea, particularly with the first few doses of an opioid.

More rare but serious side effects include:

- Sedation from the depressant effect on cells in the brainstem. Significant sedation can lead to slower breathing, which can be the first sign of an overdose.
- Misuse, which happens when a patient takes a medicine in a way not intended by the physician.

Patients occasionally experience a few other side effects. These include small muscle spasms called myoclonus, which particularly can occur as opioid doses increase; urinary retention; and reductions in levels of sex hormones. Animal studies also suggest the potential for long-term opioid therapy to cause a paradoxical hypersensitivity to pain.[7] There are also suggestions that opioids may affect the immune system, raising the risk of infection.[8] Both of these issues require further research.

Do all people who take opioids for pain develop an addiction?

No. Estimates from studies in various populations suggest that somewhere between 5% and 30% of people taking opioids for pain will develop an addiction.[9,10,11,12,13] A study from the Centers for Disease Control and Prevention assessed the chance that people who first get opioids for pain will still be taking opioids 1 or 3 years later—which is not the same as addiction. The study found that about 6% of people treated with opioids for a day were still taking opioids a year later. This rose to 27% for those whose first dose was a long-acting opioid.[14]

What are the signs of developing an addiction to opioid medications?

Preceding opioid addiction is an early stage that has been called hazardous or harmful use. These terms describe situations that are cause for concern but do not yet rise to the level of an addiction. For example, hazardous use could refer to the behavior of someone who takes opioid medications a few times in ways other than how they were prescribed. The term would also apply to someone who takes opioid pills a few times at parties with friends. It is possible that such individuals might never take extra medications or use opioids at parties again. But their behaviors nonetheless reflect a risk for developing an addiction.

The hallmarks of addiction to opioid medications are losing control over their use and continuing to use despite harmful consequences. This means taking more than prescribed, seeking the medications for their pleasurable effect, or taking the medications for reasons other than what was intended, to the point of neglecting family, work, or other social responsibilities. Obtaining and using opioids becomes the predominant focus of the person's life. The development of an addiction typically takes weeks to months after hazardous use begins. Intervention should begin as soon as problems are noticed.

How should my doctor monitor my use of opioids for pain?

Closely. For prescriptions of just a few days, doctors should prescribe the minimum necessary number of pills and be available for any questions and concerns. For ongoing pain, doctors might need to see patients every week or two (at least at first) and assess, at each visit, how the opioids are working and what side effects may be present.

Doctors should ask questions like:

- *How have you been doing since the last visit?* Your doctor should ask if you are able to go places or rejoin activities that you could not do before—or if you are becoming more socially isolated and less able to care of yourself. There are some standardized questionnaires that help doctors track function over time.[15,16] (Note that "How have you been doing?" is a better question for this purpose than "How have you been feeling?" because the latter question focuses on subjective experience rather than function.)

- *Are you constipated?* This is a good (if a bit unpleasant) initial question to start a dialogue about a range of possible side effects. Doctors should ask family members, if they are available, whether they've noticed anything unusual, such as too much sleepiness during the day.

- *How have you been taking the opioids?* This question gets at how many pills you are taking each day. It helps the doctor assess for the development of tolerance and can open the door to a discussion of misuse.

- *Can we take a look at our goals?* Your doctor should reinforce the overall plan for opioid use, including when it will be time to stop.

Before writing another prescription, your doctor may type your name into a computer that tracks all opioid prescriptions in the state or the region. This is now common practice and even law in many states. Your doctor is looking to see if you have received opioids or other controlled medications, such as sleeping pills, from other prescribers. This is important information for your doctor to have.

If I would like to reduce my use of opioid pain medications, what should I do?

When you are ready to reduce or end your use of opioids for pain, talk to your doctor. It can be very unpleasant and even dangerous to stop abruptly on your own. Your doctor will likely prescribe a schedule of gradually decreasing doses known as a taper. The Centers for Disease Control and Prevention has developed guidance for clinicians to assist with this process.[17] Some of the doses of other medications may need to be adjusted, or your doctor may recommend other types of non-medication therapies as your dose of opioids declines. If you don't feel well after reducing your dose, you should tell your doctor. It may make sense to wait a little longer before the next step down in dose.

What are signs and symptoms of an overdose from opioid medications?

All opioids cause an overdose the same way: by slowing down and eventually stopping breathing. Fortunately, there are some noticeable signs and symptoms that alert a family member or other bystander to the fact that a person is experiencing an overdose. An early sign is extreme sleepiness, with difficulty waking up. Later and very worrisome signs include gurgling or choking noises, foaming or frothing at the mouth, and lips or fingertips turning dusky or blue. A very serious sign is the inability to wake up, even when someone is causing pain by rubbing their knuckles against the breast bone in the middle of the chest. Any of these symptoms represents a medical emergency. In such situations, bystanders should administer naloxone and call 911.

Should I have naloxone on hand if I am taking an opioid medication for pain?

Yes. Naloxone is a medication that reverses opioid overdoses. Bystanders administer naloxone through an injection or a liquid squirted in the nose. The Centers for Disease Control recommends that anyone taking opioids for pain for 3 months or more have naloxone on hand at home. The American Medical Association and the Centers for Disease Control recommend that doctors consider prescribing naloxone to all patients taking opioids, taking into account such factors as the dose and history of overdose.[18,19]

Of course, it's not enough just to have naloxone somewhere in your home. Somebody has to be there, find the naloxone, and use it. Simple training on how to use naloxone is available online.[20] Talking to your parent, son, daughter, or neighbor about saving your life with naloxone is not the easiest conversation in the world. But it might be one of the most important.

Where should I store opioid medications at home?

Storage of opioid medications should be thought of the same way as storage of household cleaning supplies; the products should be accessible for their valid purpose but inaccessible to those who might misuse them. That's why it's a bad idea to leave medication vials open or keep them in easily accessed places. Some experts recommend that patients not keep opioid medications in their medicine cabinet. That's because the medicine cabinet is the first place someone searching for opioids in your home will look. A better choice would be a locked safe at home or another place others cannot access.

What should I do if I have opioid pills left over?

Get rid of your unused opioids. Fast. More than 50% of the prescription opioids misused in the United States are obtained from relatives or friends.[21]

Sharing your opioid medications with others is a particularly bad idea. Not only is it illegal, but it could make the other person's misuse of opioids worse. Far better to refer them to a physician for assessment and care. Other unsafe practices include leaving opioid medication bottles in medicine cabinets or on top of dressers, storing opioid medications in the refrigerator, mixing opioid tablets in with other medications in a pill bottle, and taking opioid pills out of their original containers and forgetting what they are.

There are a number of ways to get rid of leftover opioid pills. One of the simplest is to flush them down the toilet. The FDA publishes a list of opioids that can be safely flushed; almost all opioids are on the list.[22] While some people worry about the environmental consequences, these are minimal; after all, if you had taken the opioids, you would have urinated into the toilet about the same amount of opioid byproducts.

You can also toss the opioids in the trash. The FDA recommends mixing unwanted tablets or capsules as they are with unpalatable materials such as kitty litter or coffee grounds in a closed container, such as a plastic bag and disposing of the container in the trash. You can then delete all your personal information from the bottle label and dispose of the vial separately.[23]

Want more options? Walmart recently partnered with a company to distribute a chemical compound that, when added to a medication bottle, forms a non-toxic, gooey paste that breaks down the opioid so the whole bottle can be safely disposed in a regular trash can.[24] There are other similar products on the market.[25]

Some localities and states are designating specific drop-off sites for unwanted medication; these can be at police stations or pharmacies. The federal government and partners around the country also hold occasional medication "take back" days where people can bring their unwanted medication to a designated location for disposal.

Finally, some opioids, such as the buprenorphine patch, come with a disposal kit as part of the dispensed medication.

Why do people keep unused opioids at home?

The main reason is fear—fear that one day the pain might come back. Such a concern is understandable, but it is not a good reason to keep opioids at home when they are no longer needed. Much better to discuss with your doctor what to do if the pain recurs. A conversation and a plan can provide the confidence needed to dispose of unused medications.

3

MISUSE OF OPIOIDS

What is misuse of opioids?

Use of opioids outside of legitimate medical care is illegal in the United States. The medical and public health term for this is misuse. Misuse takes many forms and can involve stolen pills, counterfeit pills, bags of heroin, and combinations of opioids with other drugs, such as heroin mixed with cocaine.

When people misuse prescription medications, such as OxyContin®, the primary risk stems from the opioids themselves. Medications manufactured by pharmaceutical companies to exacting standards are unlikely to be contaminated. However, when people misuse counterfeit drugs, they face additional risks. These products often contain other, unknown ingredients—including the synthetic opioid fentanyl. Counterfeits may also contain an array of "fillers" that can pose threats of their own. It can be difficult to tell the difference between prescription drugs and counterfeits, which can be pressed and stamped into copycat tablets in illegal laboratories. The pop star Prince, for example, died of a fentanyl overdose after taking counterfeit prescription opioids.[1]

Some opioids—including heroin and more than 30 varieties of fentanyl—have no recognized medical use in the United States. These opioids are listed by the US Drug Enforcement Administration in Schedule I.[2] It is illegal to manufacture, possess, import, or distribute these chemicals anywhere in the United States, meaning even research with these chemicals is virtually impossible to conduct. Nonetheless, they are available through illicit markets.

When people buy these opioids on the street or over the Internet, the rule is buyer beware. As a way to make drug supplies stretch farther, dealers often cut heroin with caustic material such as talcum powder. Heroin is increasingly being mixed with illicit fentanyl or other sedating medications such as benzodiazepines that significantly increase the risk of overdose.

Misuse of opioids is dangerous for all these reasons, as well as one more: Misuse is associated with opioid addiction—a condition characterized by the loss of control over opioid use despite harmful consequences.

What are the different ways people misuse opioids?

Some people who misuse opioids swallow pills. But most misuse involves snorting, injection, or inhalation, because these methods deliver opioids to the brain faster.

Snorting

Prescription medications can be crushed and snorted. Heroin and other illicit opioids are often snorted as well. When used this way, opioids pass through the nasal tissues into the bloodstream before moving quickly to the brain. At the same time, the damage to the nasal tissues can be severe—especially when snorting heroin and other substances mixed with caustic chemicals. Some people end up with large holes in the cartilage that separates their nostrils, known as the nasal septum.

Injection

Many people suffering from addiction "graduate" from taking pills to snorting and then to injection. Injecting drugs multiple times a day takes a profound toll on the human body. Vein and skin scarring is common. Over time, as good veins for injecting become harder to find, people mistakenly inject drugs directly into their skin, leading to painful abscesses and other skin infections. This can create a vicious cycle with the person injecting again and again to relieve the pain. Because illicit drugs are not sterile, injecting them can cause serious and life-threatening bacterial infections inside the human body, including in the heart, bones, and spinal cord.

Another major risk of injection is infection from sharing supplies. Many infectious diseases, including HIV, hepatitis B and hepatitis C, are transmitted from person to person through the sharing of syringes, needles, and other equipment. The hepatitis C virus can actually survive for up to 7 days in the water used for injecting, putting people at risk for infection even if they are using their own sterile needles and syringes.

Skin popping

When there are no veins left for injection, some people resort to what is called "skin popping." Skin popping essentially is injecting directly underneath the skin. The person pinches a small piece of skin and injects into the tented area. With this method, heroin takes about 3 to 5 minutes to take effect as opposed to the 15 to 30 seconds it takes by the intravenous route. Skin popping can lead to severe infections of the skin and underlying tissues.

Inhalation

Some people who use heroin prefer to smoke it, even though some of the drug is lost in the process. Smoking heroin is called "chasing the dragon." This method involves heating the heroin, usually on a piece of aluminum foil with a lighter, and inhaling the fumes with a small tube or straw. The person using looks like he or she is "chasing" the fumes. Worldwide, inhaled heroin has overtaken injection as a primary route of use in many places. For example, nearly 3 in 4 people using heroin in Norway and 9 in 10 in Sri Lanka inhale. The practice is on the rise in the United States as well.[3] Smoking heroin has been seen as safer than injecting. However, smoking heroin can lead to seizures, strokes, and a potentially fatal type of brain damage called toxic leukoencephalopathy.

What is fentanyl?

Fentanyl is a highly potent opioid that is highly useful in medical treatment and very dangerous when misused. The pharmaceutical version of fentanyl has a variety of applications in medical care. Anesthesiologists may use this medication to reduce pain and induce sleep in the operating room. Oncologists may prescribe fentanyl lozenges for patients with severe pain from cancer.

In recent years, however, underground laboratories in China, Mexico, and elsewhere have been making illicit fentanyl and an array of compounds similar to fentanyl and selling them at low prices to dealers in the United States. These chemicals have contaminated the illicit drug supply in many areas of the United States.

People selling or buying drugs may not be aware of the presence of fentanyl. Looking for heroin? What's for sale might be heroin mixed with fentanyl, or just fentanyl. Cocaine? Could be a mixture, or just fentanyl. Prescription pills? Could be counterfeits with fentanyl. People who seek treatment for opioid addiction commonly report taking what they thought were prescription opioid pills, only to find out that they had taken fentanyl that had been compressed and stamped to look like Percocet® or OxyContin®.

This rise of fentanyl and its related compounds is causing a wave of overdoses. Illicitly manufactured fentanyl is extremely potent, typically 50 to 100 times more potent than morphine. Some of the related compounds, such as carfentanil, or the "elephant tranquilizer," may be even more potent. Others, such as cyclopropylfentanyl, have no legitimate uses in animals or humans and may bring other toxicities. Only a few grains of these chemicals can cause an overdose.

How do people start misusing opioids?

There are several paths to the misuse of opioids.

Some people start with opioid medications prescribed by their doctors, begin to misuse them, and become addicted. These people may then turn to illicit sources of opioids for several reasons. Their physicians may stop prescribing the pills, without referring them to treatment. Or they may run out of the prescribed pills early and, unable to get another refill, buy more pills from illicit sources. Or their craving for a more intense experience may be overwhelming so they turn to more potent pills sold on the street or illicit opioids such as heroin.

Other people find their way to opioid misuse through years of alcohol and marijuana use. Drug use can start early in life, particularly when people use drugs to cover up negative emotions from trauma experienced as children or to relieve psychiatric conditions such as depression. A landmark study of adverse childhood experiences found that almost 60% of adults born between 1948 and 1978 who reported 5 or more traumatic episodes as children had used an illicit drug at some point in their mid-adolescence or adulthood.[4] Alcohol and marijuana are frequently misused during the teenage years, with some people progressing to opioids either during this time or after they become adults.

Still others may misuse opioids as a result of peer pressure, not realizing that they have genetic or other biological predispositions to developing an opioid addiction. Their friends might be able to experiment with heroin and other opioids from time to time without long-lasting effect. But individuals with risk factors for addiction may use just once and feel immediately that their life has been altered forever.

All told, between 2000 and 2010, 3 out of 4 people who started using heroin had started by misusing prescription medications.[5] Evidence from more recent years, however, suggests that by 2015, larger percentages of new users were bypassing prescription opioids and going straight to heroin.[6]

Why is opioid misuse linked to risky sexual behavior?

Opioid misuse and sex have a troubled relationship. Misuse of opioids distorts perception and judgment. An intoxicated state is not ideal for remembering to wear a condom or to use other forms of birth control. As a result, opioid misuse is linked to unwanted pregnancy as well as to sexually transmitted infections, including chlamydia, gonorrhea, syphilis, and HIV.[7] Without other options for income, some men and women trade sex for drugs or sell sex for the money to buy drugs.

Why do people misuse opioids with other substances?

People who misuse opioids often misuse other substances too. Sometimes this is to intensify the feeling they get from the opioids, through a practice called "boosting." For example, some people crush and snort sedatives, like benzodiazepines (such as Xanax®), to boost the sedating, euphoric feeling of heroin. Other substances with sedating properties that are often used for boosting include alcohol; clonidine, a blood pressure medicine; quetiapine, an antidepressant often prescribed for sleep; and promethazine, an anti-nausea medication. For example, the concoction known as "purple drank" combines cough syrup that contains promethazine with the opioid codeine, as well as candy, soda, and alcohol.[8]

Sometimes people use multiple drugs to counter certain effects of the opioids. For example, some inject the stimulant cocaine with heroin together in what is known as a "speedball." In some drug markets, dealers cater to consumer preferences by mixing other substances with opioids prior to sale.

What can people who misuse opioids do to reduce their risks?

Effective treatment reduces the risk of overdose, infectious disease, other medical complications, and death. It also helps people put their lives back together.

However, some people who misuse opioids are not interested in treatment. They can very much benefit from a variety of other interventions to reduce their risks of overdose and other negative health consequences. These strategies can keep them alive until they are able to stop misusing opioids.

The strategies include:

- Using opioids with other people, with naloxone on hand in case of overdose.
- Starting with small "tester" doses of illicit drugs, to better spot products adulterated with fentanyl and related compounds.
- Using test strips to detect the presence of fentanyl directly.
- Recognizing that even a few days off of opioids (such as after an arrest) means a loss of tolerance, so smaller doses should be used if the person returns to use.
- Not sharing syringes and other supplies, not even the water used for injecting. People can go to local syringe exchange programs to obtain hygienic supplies.
- Not mixing alcohol and other sedating medications or substances with opioids. If people are going to drink or use these other substances, or even take prescribed medications, spacing the use of the opioids 2 to 3 hours apart from these other sedating substances may lessen the overdose risk.

Some people believe that programs teaching these techniques tacitly encourage illicit drug use and make it less likely for people with addiction to seek treatment. This is not the case. Studies have demonstrated that these services do not increase drug use.[9,10]

What they really do is serve as a pathway to self-care, and ultimately, to treatment. Helping people reach these programs demonstrates care for the health and lives of people with addiction, who are still husbands and wives, sisters and brothers, parents and children. With this care comes a relationship that can be a port in the storm of addiction.

4

OPIOID ADDICTION

What causes opioid addiction?

Just like it is true that not everyone who smokes will develop lung cancer, it is true that not everyone who takes or even misuses an opioid will develop an opioid addiction. While the biology of opioid addiction is still under investigation, research has identified several different factors that contribute to the development of addiction.

Individual factors

Genetic risk accounts for about 40% to 60% of the risk of developing an addiction. For opioid addiction, it is likely that the involved genes relate to opioid receptors, to the brain pathways involved in reward and pleasure, and to pathways not yet fully understood.[1]

A clue to the genetics of opioids can be seen in their side effects. About one-third of people who take a dose of codeine or morphine for the first time experience nausea and vomiting, which leads them to not take any more. This group of people have a lower risk of developing an opioid addiction compared to others.

Another individual risk factor for addiction is immaturity. The part of the brain that controls judgment, the prefrontal cortex, is the last part of the brain to mature. That's why many teenagers and young adults impulsively do dangerous things, including misusing substances, without seeming to think about the risks. Other risk factors include the presence of other mental health conditions particularly mood disorders and schizophrenia; a history of trauma, especially early child-hood trauma; and exposure to substances before age 14. In fact, people with significant histories of adverse childhood experiences have almost 8 times the chance of developing an addiction compared to individuals without any such life events.[2]

The environment

The greater the availability of opioids, the greater chance for addiction. A major reason for the recent opioid epidemic is the large increase in the amount of opioids prescribed for pain. As opioid medications began to appear in medicine cabinets across the country, opportunities for misuse and addiction multiplied.

Neighborhood conditions contribute substantially to risk. Communities suffering from extreme poverty and joblessness experience more addiction to opioids; this may be a function of greater levels of despair, which leads people to turn to substances for escape from their daily circumstances. It also may relate to relatively greater avail-ability of opioids in these neighborhoods and less access to effective treatment.

The opioids themselves

Opioids that are high potency and able to reach the brain quickly through injection, snorting, or inhalation are more likely to lead to addiction than others that are usually taken by mouth. For example, someone who injects heroin is more likely to develop an opioid addiction than someone who swallows a dose of codeine.

What is happening in the brain of someone with an opioid addiction?

Deep in the reward center of the brain of someone with addiction, an opioid causes—at least at first—an enormous release of the neurotransmitter dopamine. The result is an intense feeling of pleasure, warmth, and well-being. Some patients with opioid addiction have described it as being wrapped in the warmest, most comforting blanket in the world, like a gigantic bear hug. Others have said that there was a serene numbness that came over them so that even though they were still in physical or emotional pain or distress, it did not really matter anymore.

For a while, the brain's reward center can continue producing high levels of dopamine. But with every use, the amount of dopamine released declines, and the intensity of the response diminishes. By this time, however, the brain circuits of reward, motivation, learning, and memory have been hijacked; the usual sources of pleasure do not matter. At the same time that the deep parts of the brain are in a ramped-up drive to produce dopamine, they effectively become uncoupled from the part of the brain that controls awareness and exerts impulse control, known as the pre-frontal cortex. So the part of the brain that could exert a brake on the compulsive drive that keeps people using is not able to do so. What matters now to the addicted brain are the things—people, places, objects, smells, and emotions—that are associated with using opioids. "Triggers" is the word commonly used to describe these environmental and psychological cues to using.

As intense opioid use continues, the brain adapts. The number and responsiveness of opioid receptors declines, in effect protecting the brain from high levels of stimulation. A "new normal" sets in that depends on external sources of opioids; the individual's own endorphins are not nearly enough to generate feelings of pleasure or even of equanimity. The result is a need for opioids to avoid a state of distress and negative emotions.

These changes often contribute to social isolation, just at the time when people need the most assistance to change.

What are triggers?

Triggers are all the cues, both internal and external, that, over time, become associated in the brain with the use of opioids and the anticipated feelings of pleasure and reward. Triggers range from people, places, and things to smells, stress, and both extremely positive and negative internal emotional states. These become drivers of impulsive, ongoing use in people with opioid addiction.

Here's a case example: A 27-year-old man who had been using heroin and cocaine for 10 years starts treatment with buprenorphine, moves into a recovery house, and stabilizes his opioid and cocaine addiction. He then relapses to cocaine use, is very upset with himself, and doesn't know what to do. He sees his doctor, who says, "Tell me exactly what you did yesterday, from the minute you woke up in the morning to the moment you went to bed." The young man slowly starts to recount his day, noting that he got up as usual, felt fine, ate breakfast, and left the house with all the other men to walk the three blocks to the treatment center where he was expected for a group counseling session. As he describes walking down the street, his eyes suddenly widen, and he draws his breath. "I've got it!" he yells out. "They're paving the street!" He then explains that smell of the tar being used to pave a street near his house reminds him of the smell of his cocaine, which he heated before injecting. They discuss a plan for him to take an alternate route from the house to the center to avoid the triggering smell. One week later, he returns to see the doctor and proudly announces that he has not used any cocaine since implementing the alternative route and has added "tar smell" to the list of triggers he keeps on a piece of paper in his wallet.

What are drug dreams?

Drug dreams are extremely vivid dreams of drug use and euphoria that occur even after someone has stopped the misuse of opioids. Drug dreams are thought to occur as a function of the human brain's capacity to absorb an enormous amount of information through sight, smell, taste, touch, and hearing. Triggers not previously recognized by the awake and conscious brain may set off such intense drug dreams that a person may wake up wondering out loud if she had just used heroin again after many years in remission and recovery. Walking people through their 24 hours prior to the dream can often help them identify what the trigger was. With such awareness, future cravings associated with those triggers can be recognized and managed in a healthy way.

Here's a case example: A 42-year-old man comes to see his doctor for his monthly visit to check his blood pressure and obtain a prescription for buprenorphine. When asked about cravings or drug dreams he may have had in the last month, he hesitatingly says, "Yeah, I had a weird dream the other night. I've never had drug dreams before so I'm not sure what to make of it." He goes on to describe the dream as feeling himself getting high on heroin in a house where he lived a decade earlier. He woke up in a sweat, wondering if he had indeed just done what he had worked so hard not to do for the past 3 years. When the doctor points out to him that drug dreams signal that his brain has been triggered by something, he sits up and says:

> I know what it is. The son of a woman who lived in the house that appeared in my dream called recently to tell me he had found a picture of me and his mother. She just passed away a few months ago, so I've been thinking about her a lot. I went to the house to pick up the picture. It's weird; the moment I stepped across the door jamb to the front door, I felt that same bubbling sensation in my

stomach that I used to get just before I used heroin. My palms got all sweaty. So I didn't stay long. The craving went away as soon as I left the house. I thought I was done with it after that.

Is opioid addiction a disease?

Yes. Someone with opioid addiction has impaired brain function that causes a characteristic set of symptoms—the very definition of disease. The Merriam-Webster dictionary's definition states that a disease can be caused by "environmental factors" as well as matters "inherent" to the organism.[3] The disease of addiction involves contributions from both the environment and the individual.

Surveys indicate, however, that only a slim majority of Americans agree with calling addiction a disease.[4] Others describe addiction as a choice, a moral failure, or a crime. Arguments against calling opioid addiction a disease fall into three categories.

- *"People choose to use drugs, at least the first time. Something can't be a disease if it starts with a voluntary action."*

   Not true. Lung cancer almost always results from smoking cigarettes, and diabetes often results from overeating and obesity. Even the common cold might be said to originate with behavior. People make decisions, after all, not to wash their hands as often as they should.
- *"They can stop at any time. It's not possible to stop a disease."*

   This perspective confuses the disease (brain dysfunction) for an action (taking the drug). In fact, these are separable. Even when someone is able to stop, their brain is still affected, and the person may suffer from significant craving and other symptoms.

   People who are unaffected by addiction often think, "If it were me, I would be rational and choose to stop using right away." But addiction interferes with the capacity to exert rational control. Why would someone choose to continue to use even after almost dying several times? Why would someone choose to suffer from blistering, painful, infected abscesses on her arms and legs? Why would anyone want to lose his job, his family, his home? The answer can be found in the dysfunction affecting their brains.

- *"Calling addiction a disease means there is no personal responsibility."*

Many people object to calling addiction a disease on the grounds that doing so excuses an individual of responsibility. In fact, people with a disease, especially a chronic one, have a critical responsibility—to manage their condition.

For example, when the body's cells become resistant to insulin, the resulting disease is called diabetes. Yet the biology is just the beginning. To avoid or delay severe complications, such as blindness and kidney failure, people with diabetes must change how they shop for food, how they cook, and how and what they eat. They must exercise regularly. Many find that managing their disease leads them to restructure their lives. Yet, despite this enormous role for personal responsibility, everyone recognizes that diabetes is a disease.

In the same way, without removing the role of personal responsibility, it is possible to see opioid addiction as a disease. Like patients with diabetes, people with opioid addiction must restructure their lives to avoid terrible complications. This may start with regular visits to a syringe services program or to an outreach worker, progress to treatment at a local clinic, and conclude with a series of life changes required for recovery. Individuals with opioid addiction must accept their illness, learn as much as they can about the way it affects them, and figure out how to live with it, and despite it.

How do doctors diagnose opioid addiction?

Addiction is a clinical diagnosis, meaning that health-care practitioners diagnose the condition based on specific symptoms, or diagnostic criteria. There is no X-ray, computed tomography (CT) scan, or blood test to make the diagnosis of an opioid use disorder, the condition that reflects an addiction. While some people think that a positive drug test is all that is needed, that is not the case.

These diagnostic criteria can be found in a book called the *Diagnostic and Statistical Manual, Version 5 (DSM-5)*, published by the American Psychiatric Association. To meet the diagnosis of opioid use disorder, a patient has to meet at least 2 of the 11 symptoms, or diagnostic criteria, for this condition. A person having 6 or more symptoms at the time the diagnosis is made has a severe opioid use disorder.

The 11 symptoms in the *DSM-5* are:

1. Taking the substance in larger amounts or for longer than intended.
2. Wanting to cut down or stop using the substance but not being able to.
3. Spending a lot of time getting, using, or recovering from use of the substance.
4. Cravings and urges to use the substance.
5. Not managing to do what you should at work, home, or school because of substance use.
6. Continuing to use, even when it causes problems in relationships.
7. Giving up important social, occupational, or recreational activities because of substance use.
8. Using substances again and again, even when it puts you in danger.
9. Continuing to use, even when you know you have a physical or psychological problem that could have been caused or made worse by the substance.

10. Needing more of the substance to get the effect you want (tolerance).
11. Development of withdrawal symptoms, which can be relieved by taking more of the substance.[5]

There is one important point in the *DSM-5*: the last two criteria alone, tolerance and withdrawal, are not sufficient to make the diagnosis of opioid use disorder in a patient appropriately taking opioid medications. See Appendix 5 for further details.

What are the consequences of opioid addiction?

Left untreated, opioid addiction is a devastating disease. Opioid addiction often leads to profound social isolation, as individuals lose their employment, families, and homes. Those who commit crimes to obtain opioids frequently pass in and out of the criminal justice system.

Medical complications depend in part on the type of opioid use. For example, people who snort opioids can suffer perforations in nasal passages, and individuals who inject opioids can develop skin abscesses, heart valve infections, HIV, and hepatitis C. Then there is the serious risk of fatal overdose.

How long does opioid addiction last?

As a chronic disease that affects the brain, opioid addiction lasts a long time, with a potential risk of relapse even after extended periods of stability. That's the bad news.

The good news is that many individuals achieve sustained remission and recovery. Every year in recovery reduces the risk of relapse. Once 3 to 5 years have passed, the risk drops below 15%.[6] Many people with opioid addiction reconnect with their families, find jobs, and live their lives with meaning and purpose. Even those who relapse are often able to re-engage in treatment and achieve a more durable recovery.

Do people with addiction want to stop using opioids?

Yes. Very often, people with an opioid addiction want to stop using. Having an opioid addiction is painful, both emotionally and physically. Losing control of one's life, coming close to dying from an overdose, and all the other negative consequences of an addiction is not something people ever want or envision for themselves. However, the disease is such that the desire to stop using is often fleeting. It can be pushed aside by fear of withdrawal, craving for a high, and the opportunity to use again. That's why it's critical to make opportunities for services and treatment as readily available as possible.

5

OPIOID OVERDOSE

What affects the risk of opioid overdose?

Several factors influence the risk of overdose from opioids, including a person's level of tolerance; the amount, potency, and type of the opioid taken; age; other medical conditions; and the presence of other sedating substances or medications.

The threshold at which an overdose occurs varies by person. A person who has never taken an opioid before will overdose more readily than a person who has been taking opioids for a long time. In general, older people are more likely to die from overdose than younger people. This is because older livers and older kidneys have a more difficult time eliminating opioids from the body. People with obstructive sleep apnea are at high risk of opioid overdose, because they already have physical changes inhibiting their breathing at night.

Combining opioids with alcohol, medications in the benzodiazepine family, such as diazepam (Valium®) and alprazolam (Xanax®), and other sedatives increases the risk of overdose. The effects of multiple substances are greater than any one alone. Alcohol also may disrupt the extended-release properties of some opioid formulations, causing a rapid release of a large amount of opioids in the stomach and intestines all at once.[1]

Two characteristics of opioids themselves particularly influence the risk of overdose. One is the potency. For example, just a tiny amount of fentanyl can stop breathing, so fentanyl is associated with a high risk of overdose. That is why doctors should not prescribe fentanyl to patients who have not developed a tolerance to opioids.

A second characteristic is the extent to which the opioid, when bound to a receptor, fully activates nerve cells in the brainstem. For example, because the medication buprenorphine only partially activates these cells, it carries a lower overdose risk than other types of opioids.

How can I tell if someone is experiencing an opioid overdose?

All opioids cause an overdose the same way: by slowing down and eventually stopping breathing. An early sign is extreme sleepiness and difficulty in waking up. Later and very worrisome signs include gurgling or choking noises, foaming or frothing at the mouth, a dusky or blue color to lips or fingertips, and an inability to arouse—even when someone else rubs their knuckles against the person's breast bone in the middle of the chest. When these symptoms occur, it is a medical emergency. It's time to give naloxone and call 911.

What should I do if I suspect someone is experiencing an opioid overdose?

Respond quickly! First, rub your knuckles firmly against the person's breastbone in the middle of the chest. This hurts. So if the person is just sleeping, they should wake up and demand to know what you're doing. (You were just being concerned.)

Second, call for assistance. This can be as simple as asking someone else to call 911.

Third, if you have naloxone, use it. Naloxone can be delivered by injection into a large muscle, such as the front of the thigh; the needle can be pushed right through the person's clothing. If you have a liquid or spray form of naloxone, squeeze a dose up the nose.

If you do not have naloxone at hand and you have been trained in basic life support, the American Heart Association recommends providing 2 minutes of cardiopulmonary resuscitation (CPR), if needed, before leaving the victim to find naloxone.[2]

Once the person wakes up and begins to breathe more regularly, roll the person onto his or her side. This reduces the chance of choking on saliva and other secretions.

If the person has used fentanyl, it is possible multiple doses of naloxone may be needed, with about 2 to 4 minutes in between each one. When emergency medical personnel give naloxone, about 1 in 6 people need more than one dose.[3]

If still no response, it is possible the person may not be experiencing an opioid overdose at all. It could be an overdose of another substance, such as alcohol or cocaine, or something else altogether, such as a stroke or a heart attack. In these situations, naloxone will not work, and first responders will need to assess for other problems.

What are the different forms of naloxone and how are they used?

Naloxone comes in three formulations.

A liquid vial

The liquid can be drawn into a syringe and injected into the muscle, into a vein, or in the subcutaneous layer just under the skin. It also can be used with a syringe or spray nozzle and administered through the nose. This form of naloxone is off-patent, but the companies that make it have increased the price in recent years. In 2018, this formulation cost about $35 per vial.[4]

A liquid vial already connected to a spray nozzle, known as an "intranasal applicator"

This formulation is approved by the Food and Drug Administration for use through the nose. This formulation, known as Narcan®, is under patent; in 2018, the company made it available to governments for $75 for two vials.[5]

An auto-injector

This device speaks using a recorded voice command. The voice walks the rescuer through the 3-step process of injecting naloxone. This formulation, known as Evzio™, is also under patent, with the manufacturer receiving criticism in recent years for raising the price to several thousand dollars a dose.[6]

What happens after someone suffering an opioid overdose gets naloxone?

Signs of a response to naloxone start to appear within seconds, and the person is usually alert within a couple of minutes.

The reason for this life-saving effect? Naloxone reverses the effects of opioids on the brain. Naloxone reverses all the other effects opioids have on the body too, triggering a withdrawal syndrome. So, instead of constipation from opioids, the person now may develop diarrhea. Other common reactions to naloxone include nausea, vomiting, profuse sweating, severe runny eyes, runny nose, and body aches. These reactions will be strongest among people who have developed a tolerance to opioids prior to overdosing.

And if someone was using an opioid for a pleasurable sensation, that's gone too. In its place is often irritability and agitation.

People who have just received naloxone are usually alive and awake but not particularly happy. People whose lives have been saved may even express anger, rather than gratitude, toward their rescuers. This response, understandably, can be upsetting. But, it is important to remember that this initial reaction is due to discomfort and pain. Later on, many who experience overdose are extremely grateful to those who have saved their lives.

Do I still need to call 911 if I have rescued someone with naloxone?

Yes. Someone who had stopped breathing because of opioids will breathe on their own for as long as the naloxone stays in the body. If the naloxone wears off before the opioid does, the person may stop breathing again. So getting people to medical care as soon as possible is important.

How can I get naloxone?

Talk to your local pharmacist. In many places, there is a standing order for naloxone, meaning that anyone can get a dose.[7] If there is no standing order in your area, your pharmacist may direct you to your doctor or to public health agencies that may be holding trainings and distributing doses directly.

6

TREATMENT FOR OPIOID ADDICTION

What are the goals of treatment for opioid addiction?

The three major goals of treatment are to stay alive, to reduce and then stop opioid misuse, and to begin to rebuild a life.

Amid an epidemic of opioid overdoses, staying alive is a goal for everyone with opioid addiction. In the initial phases of treatment, when many people continue to misuse opioids and other harmful substances, this goal is paramount. It is not uncommon for misuse to continue off and on as people learn how to manage the triggers they face in their daily lives.

With time, a primary focus of treatment shifts to helping people stop misusing opioids entirely. Some people reach this stage within days; others, within weeks to months. (This can be a particularly rewarding moment for clinicians, who have watched someone move from despair and the brink of death to action and hope.) As the brains and bodies of persons with addiction stabilize, so do their lives. Individuals at this stage are in remission and no longer experiencing the harmful consequences of continued opioid use.

Here's a case example: A 52-year-old woman who has been using heroin for the past 20 years walks into a treatment program for help. She has experienced 2 overdoses in the past 6 months, each time revived with naloxone. Her husband threatened divorce after the last overdose. She works full-time in a local school cafeteria and wants to apply for a manager position. She has been late a couple of times for work because of car trouble, but spent the money for the repairs on heroin. She starts treatment with buprenorphine and weekly outpatient therapy but needs an additional 6 weeks of intensive counseling services to stabilize. She and her husband get back together. Together, they pull together enough money to get her car fixed. She wants to not be late for even one day of work.

The next goal is to achieve recovery. This process has been characterized as a time of personal growth and a striving for meaning and purpose in life. For one person, recovery may involve reconciling with her children and embracing her role as grandmother; for another person, the goal may be getting his job back and moving up in his company; still another may focus on restarting her education to pursue her dream of becoming a teacher. At this point, clinicians and patients together should broaden the treatment plan to include a recovery plan and to identify resources that can help that plan become a reality.

Here's a case example: A 38-year-old man seeks help for a 15-year battle with heroin. The battle has cost him his marriage and left him with hepatitis C, a life-threatening infection of the liver. Once in treatment with methadone, he finds that his cravings for heroin have disappeared, and he is able to focus on rebuilding his life. A decade later, he is happily remarried, has two children, and owns his own furniture business, which employs 30 people. A course of antiviral medication has cured his hepatitis C infection. He returns to the treatment program once a month to pick up his methadone, check in with his counselor, and see his doctor as needed.

What are effective ways to engage people with opioid addiction in treatment?

In the 1990s, researchers developed an approach to smoking cessation that has since been applied to a number of chronic diseases, including opioid addiction.[1] This approach recognizes that some people have no interest in change, while others are considering taking important steps forward but have yet to follow through. The major insight from this model is that the best response to someone depends on their mindset at the moment.

Not interested in stopping misuse of opioids

Many people with opioid addiction refuse to seek assistance, thinking they do not need help.[2] This state of mind may be a symptom of their disease, but other factors contribute as well. For some people, admitting a problem undermines how they want to see themselves. Others have lost loved ones to overdose and cannot bear the thought of being at risk for the same fate. Still others have had negative or traumatic past experiences with treatment. An unhelpful term for people in this stage is "denial." "Denial" obscures the real reasons why people are reluctant to see their addiction as a problem.

People who are uninterested in changing their drug use often engender strong feelings of frustration and despair in others. The problem is so obvious to friends and family members. So how could it not be to the person with the addiction? Unfortunately, this is the nature of addiction: compulsive craving and use no matter the consequences.

At this stage, the key goal is safety. Ordering people to go to a treatment program is often not very effective, especially if the treatment program has rigid rules. Even if people with the addiction initially go along with such a plan, they often leave, abscond, or relapse, making it seem as if the person failed or the treatment was ineffective. In reality, the intervention did not match the mindset of the person with the disease.

A better approach is to help people at this stage access harm reduction services, such as naloxone distribution and syringe services. These programs not only reduce the risk of death and other consequences, but they also establish a human connection. Staff in harm reduction programs can help people to recognize the benefits of treatment and make a referral to care.

Here's a case example: An 18-year-old man who was traumatized in his childhood by sexual abuse and consumed alcohol and marijuana heavily begins using heroin. His practice is to inject heroin together with cocaine with a set of friends from high school. Despite his history and risky behaviors, he visits a syringe services program regularly and learns how to avoid infectious diseases. As a result, he never suffers from an abscess, a heart infection, HIV, or hepatitis C. After several years, he accepts a referral from syringe services staff to treatment.

Considering stopping misuse of opioids

For some people, accepting there is a problem makes things "click" into place once and for all. They not only sign up for treatment but also make wholesale changes in how they respond to triggers, whom they befriend, how they spend their time, where they go, and how they deal with negative feelings. For many others, however, the transition from active use to successful treatment passes through a stage known as "contemplation."

In this stage, people with opioid addiction recognize they have a problem but still feel ambivalent about change. They may sign up for treatment, while continuing to misuse drugs. This paradox reflects the fact that the brain dysfunction associated with addiction does not resolve all at once. The reward and other brain circuits involved in addiction lie in the subconscious part of the brain, often functioning and responding to external and internal cues automatically. As a result, it is common for people with addiction to ask for help to stop one minute—and mean it—and the next minute, to disappear in search of drugs.

During the time that people are contemplating stopping their misuse, their desire to change should be reinforced and supported by all of those around them. In particular, their clinicians at treatment programs should recognize that the early phases of care can be marked by fits and starts. The goal at this stage is to help the person overcome ambivalence and commit to change.

Here's a case example: A 32-year-old man who had been snorting prescription opioids since his early 20s comes with his mother to her doctor's office. The young man has been in and out of several expensive residential treatment facilities, every time receiving a brief course of medications to temporarily treat his withdrawal symptoms. After each episode of treatment, he returns to a stressful job and an apartment he shares with his girlfriend of 10 years. She uses cocaine and does not contribute to the rent.

Now the young man says he decided over a Christmas vacation at home that he is ready for treatment again. The mother's physician takes him on as a patient and prescribes buprenorphine. The next day, however, the young man returns to his apartment and girlfriend, throws away the buprenorphine, and snorts several oxycodone tablets. Two months later, he returns to the doctor. In describing what happened, the young man says, "I felt really stressed having to go to work that day, even after taking a dose of the medication. My boss has been really good to me and the people I work with are nice, but I hate the job. But what choice do I have since I'm the only one paying the rent? The oxycodone at least makes it kind of bearable."

Over the next couple of months, figuring out how to deal with the girlfriend and the job and taking buprenorphine consistently become the focus of the treatment plan for the patient, the doctor, and the patient's counselor. The patient misses another couple of appointments as a result of relapse but ultimately comes back, takes his medication every day and receives care for depression as well. He eventually decides to end his dysfunctional relationship with his girlfriend and finds a different job, one he likes to this day.

What is remission?

Effective treatment for opioid addiction leads to remission, a state of substantial improvement in the symptoms of addiction. Remission means no longer misusing opioids and putting the pieces of a normal life back together.

Remission is accompanied by a number of changes in the brain. The most significant is that the prefrontal cortex, which is responsible for awareness, judgment, and voluntary action, takes control over subconscious parts of the brain, including the reward pathway. Evidence is emerging that this shift is accompanied by new connections between these parts of the brain.[3]

Even in remission, however, the risk of relapse never completely goes away. Unforeseen circumstances and unappreciated triggers can disrupt the reward system. A return to misuse may occur, which can be devastating to friends and family members. Yet all is not lost. Often, the person re-engages in treatment, learns from the relapse, and takes steps to prevent the situation from happening again.

What is effective treatment for opioid addiction?

Effective treatment for opioid addiction has several components—including medication, counseling, and other supports—that, according to clinical guidelines, "should be matched to a person's needs."[4]

There are three types of medications approved by the Food and Drug Administration (FDA) for opioid addiction: methadone, buprenorphine, and naltrexone. All three work somewhat differently in the brain and body and have different side- effects. All three medications have been tested and found effective in reducing illicit opioid use, measured both by drug testing and by self-report.

There are also different kinds of counseling. Many people benefit from behavioral therapy in community settings. This can occur in group or individual sessions, lasting anywhere from an hour once a month to several hours a day. Trained healthcare practitioners, including physicians, can also provide counseling as part of medical visits. A key goal of counseling is to help people learn to recognize their triggers for opioid use and how to respond to them successfully. Counseling can also uncover some of the psychological factors contributing to addiction and how to manage them.

Most people do well in community treatment programs. A therapeutic environment such as a residential treatment center may be helpful at the start of treatment for people with severe opioid use disorder, particularly when complicated by addiction to other substances and significant social needs.

Other supports vary according to the needs of the individual. Many with opioid addiction benefit from access to mental health treatment and medical care for a variety of conditions. There are also important social needs to attend to, including safe and affordable housing, childcare, and adequate nutrition. Career counseling and employment support can help people achieve a sustainable recovery.

When is the right time to start treatment for opioid addiction?

As soon as someone is interested in treatment. Because of the nature of addiction to opioids, waiting—even for a day or two—can make it difficult for people to follow through.

Having an active addiction reflects ongoing brain dysfunction that operates subconsciously and can manifest without warning. There may only be hours to intervene before someone with addiction will start to crave opioids again and experience the onset of withdrawal. These symptoms often drive people to disappear in search of opioids, missing appointments for treatment—even those scheduled for the next morning.

Here's a case example: A married couple in their 20s walk into a treatment program with a dire story. The husband began misusing prescription opioids after he was injured at work and soon after started to share them with his wife. Once pills became too expensive, they switched to heroin. They lost their home, lost custody of their son, took to living in a tent, and began panhandling for money. Now they are asking for help. The physician immediately starts both on buprenorphine, eliminating their symptoms of withdrawal and dramatically reducing their cravings. The program also finds them safe housing. Now six years later, they work full-time, have regained custody of their son, have a new daughter, and share a household with his elderly mother.

How are the needs of someone with opioid addiction assessed?

Addiction treatment professionals often use standardized questionnaires to assess the needs of new patients. These questionnaires cover the details of past and present use of opioids and other substances, previous episodes of treatment, and other mental health and medical problems. They also cover where patients are living, what kind of work they have done, and how far they went in school. The information gathered helps the treating clinicians to identify a range of social needs and determine the best setting for care. Medical practitioners use the information to guide medication recommendations and identify other healthcare needs. Even with highly qualified professionals and electronic assessment tools, the assessment process can often take several hours to complete. The questions sometimes can go on so long that it is not uncommon for some people with opioid addiction to start feeling unwell from withdrawal.

As a result, some addiction treatment programs are moving toward doing a much briefer, medically focused assessment to start, followed by a dose of an effective treatment medication. Once the person is feeling better, either that same day or the next day, then the full assessment is much easier to complete.

Assessment is not just "one and done." Just like with diabetes or hypertension, people with opioid addiction need regular re-assessments to evaluate how they are responding to treatment—including how they are doing with the medication they are taking and the counseling services they are receiving. It is also important to find out if new needs have arisen that require attention. Re-assessments help the clinician and the patient jointly change strategies that may not be working and reinforce ones that are.

What is methadone?

Methadone is an opioid medication originally developed in Germany in the late 1930s for the treatment of pain. In the 1960s, researchers in New York City first began to study methadone as a treatment for opioid addiction.

The early results found that a single daily dose of methadone produced substantial benefits.[5] The medication not only effectively relieved the symptoms of heroin withdrawal, but it also significantly reduced heroin cravings. In addition, researchers noticed that the use of methadone in patients with heroin addiction did not cause euphoria. Methadone use normalized behavior so patients no longer committed crimes and could effectively function in society. Because methadone could be taken orally, patients no longer needed to use needles for injecting opioids, resulting in lower risks of abscesses and other infections.

Further research has identified that the key to methadone's success for addiction treatment is its long duration in the human body. A dose of methadone typically lasts 24 or 36 hours. Daily dosing leads to a steady state of medication, without the ups and downs associated with heroin and other shorter-acting opioids. Methadone also outcompetes other opioids for the opioid receptor. This characteristic means that patients who are taking methadone are less likely to overdose, even in the case of relapse to heroin, since methadone blocks much of the effect of the heroin.

To be successful, methadone must be delivered at a therapeutic dose. Unfortunately, many physicians have a mistaken belief that 60 mg per day should be the maximum dose for anyone taking methadone for the treatment of opioid addiction. Well-done studies have shown that doses between 80 and 100 mg daily are safe and much more effective at reducing illicit opioid use compared to 60 mg daily.[6] Some patients need even higher doses.

Since its introduction, dozens of studies have confirmed the benefits of methadone for the treatment of opioid addiction. It is now well established that treatment with the medication reduces illicit opioid use,[7] helps people stay in treatment longer,[8] reduces drug-related crime,[9] improves rates of employment,[10] reduces needle-sharing among injection opioid users,[11] reduces rates of HIV and hepatitis C transmission,[12,13] and improves quality of life.[14] Most important, treatment with methadone reduces opioid-related mortality by up to 80% compared with no treatment.[15]

Methadone has several important risks and side effects. For one, methadone can cause significant euphoria in people who have never taken an opioid before or who use opioids infrequently. For this reason, the federal government has designated methadone as a controlled substance and requires that methadone be reserved for patients with moderate to severe opioid addiction.

Second, methadone can cause overdose, particularly in people with low tolerance. Therefore, people keeping methadone in their homes need to lock up the medication, keep it far away from children, and not give any of it to other people (or to pets).

Third, methadone can affect part of the electrical cycle of the heart. This effect, called QT prolongation, can increase the risk of a potentially fatal heart arrhythmia called Torsade de Pointes. Electrolyte imbalances, such as too little potassium, and a host of other medications, also can cause QT prolongation. It is therefore important for patients to make their other healthcare providers aware that they are taking methadone. Healthcare practitioners can identify QT prolongation through a simple electrocardiogram (EKG) and then take steps to reduce the risk.

Fourth, because methadone is itself an opioid, someone taking the medication will develop side effects similar to other opioids, such as constipation. As with all opioids, if methadone is abruptly stopped or cut back, the person will develop withdrawal symptoms.

Does methadone make people sleepy?

At the right dose for a particular patient, methadone does not cause sleepiness. There are two reasons why methadone has a bad reputation for making people sleepy.

First, it can take some time to find the patient's correct dose. Federal law requires doctors to start with relatively low doses and then gradually increase them. This means that patients starting methadone often continue misusing other opioids. It can take several days to a couple of weeks of slowly increasing doses to get to a therapeutic dose. Because methadone is so long-acting, blood levels may continue to rise during that period and cause some sedation. It may then be necessary to lower the dose to find the optimal dose to take each day. This correct dose will not make the patient sleepy. Instead, it will reduce or eliminate cravings, suppress withdrawal, and allow the patient to function normally.

Second, people on methadone may still be misusing other substances, including benzodiazepines such diazepam (Valium®) and alprazolam (Xanax®). These combinations can cause significant sedation. Stopping the benzodiazepines should resolve the sleepiness.

If you feel sleepy on methadone, tell your doctor, who can figure out what is happening and make some changes.

Can I take other medications with methadone?

Yes, but the dose of methadone and the other medications may need to be adjusted. The enzyme system in the liver that metabolizes methadone also metabolizes many other medicines—including medications for HIV, depression, and different bacterial infections. When the liver encounters all these different medications at once, the result can be either higher or lower blood levels of methadone or of one or more of the other medicines. For example, patients taking carbamazepine for a seizure disorder metabolize methadone more quickly, requiring doctors to prescribe a larger dose to be effective.

What are opioid treatment programs?

Opioid treatment programs are outpatient clinics authorized under federal law to provide addiction treatment with methadone. These centers are highly regulated. For example, the Drug Enforcement Administration sets standards for physical security of the medications, the layout of the clinic, and procedures to guard against unauthorized use and theft. Another federal agency, the Substance Abuse and Mental Health Services Administration requires that opioid treatment programs conduct a complete history and physical exam on every patient, provide counseling, and offer a set of other services.

Regulations require that patients receiving methadone come to opioid treatment programs every day for at least the first 3 months before being considered for a couple of days of "take-home" medication. As patients stabilize, they are able to take medication home for longer periods of time. After two years, stable patients are permitted to bring up to a month's supply home at once.

Opioid treatment programs were once known as "methadone programs." However, this outdated term does not reflect the range of services that the centers offer. Many offer other types of treatment for opioid use disorder, including with FDA-approved medications other than methadone. Some opioid treatment programs now offer treatment for hepatitis C, screening and care for sexually transmitted disease, reproductive health services, and even primary care.

Every opioid treatment program has a policy on when to discharge patients from treatment. Some have strict rules and release patients who do not come for counseling or who test positive for illicit substances, even once. Others have more fully embraced the evidence for treating opioid addiction as a chronic brain disease and recognize that it may take time for someone to achieve remission and recovery. The federal Centers for Substance Abuse Treatment at the Department of Health and Human Services recommends against arbitrarily discharging patients from care,[16] for the compelling reason that discharging patients from treatment carries significant risks of relapse and overdose.

What is buprenorphine?

Buprenorphine is an opioid medication developed in the 1970s for the treatment of pain and then studied in the 1980s for the treatment of opioid addiction. The results were quite positive: fewer cravings, less illicit opioid use, and longer durations in treatment.[17] In 2000, Congress passed legislation that allowed any licensed physician, after receiving 8 hours of special training, to write prescriptions for buprenorphine for a certain number of patients to treat opioid addiction.[18]

Buprenorphine has some unique chemical properties. Like other opioids, buprenorphine attaches to opioid receptors. Unlike with other opioids, however, this binding does not activate the cell fully. This means that its impact on the respiratory center in the brainstem is less, translating into a lower risk of overdose. In fact, it is rare for someone to die from an overdose of buprenorphine alone; however, it has been implicated in some deaths in combination with benzodiazepines, such as diazepam (Valium®).

Like methadone, buprenorphine is long-acting, so one daily dose of buprenorphine is enough to suppress the withdrawal from other opioids. Buprenorphine also has a high affinity for the opioid receptor, so the medication will block the effects of other opioids that come along. For example, at a therapeutic dose of buprenorphine, the person will not feel anything from oxycodone or heroin. Patients have been known to test this blockade but typically return to the doctor saying "You were right, doc. I wasted $40 on heroin and didn't feel a thing!"

This same characteristic, however, can complicate starting treatment. Patients who have recently used heroin or other opioids can experience withdrawal symptoms upon starting buprenorphine. This effect happens because buprenorphine outcompetes all other opioids, including methadone, for the opioid receptor, and the nerve cells experience this change as a loss of activation. The technical term for this condition is "precipitated withdrawal." Patients who experience precipitated withdrawal may be reluctant to continue treatment with buprenorphine.

To avoid this problem, it is recommended that people start treatment with buprenorphine when they show signs of withdrawal.

A large number of studies have demonstrated the safety and effectiveness of buprenorphine for the treatment of opioid addiction. Buprenorphine significantly reduces use of illicit opioids,[19] keeps people in treatment,[20] dramatically reduces HIV-risk behaviors,[21] and reduces deaths from opioid overdose by about 75%.[22]

Buprenorphine can cause the same side effects, such as constipation, associated with other opioids, but these are typically not as severe. People can misuse and develop an addiction to buprenorphine, but this typically occurs in people with little previous exposure to opioids. Addiction is also less likely to occur with the most commonly used form of buprenorphine in the United States, in which buprenorphine is combined with naloxone.

Buprenorphine is sold by itself as a generic tablet, as a patch (Butrans®), as a long-term implantable (Probuphine®), and now as a month-long injection (Sublocade®). The implanted and injected forms are relatively new to the market, and additional formulations are on the horizon. These may have greater roles in clinical practice in the near future.

Why does buprenorphine come in a formulation mixed with naloxone?

Buprenorphine is most commonly available in combination with the reversal drug naloxone. The combination is available as a tablet placed under the tongue (generic as well as the brand name Zubsolv®), as a film also placed under the tongue (brand name Suboxone®), and as a film that is placed in the cheek (brand name Bunavail®). (Unlike many other medications, buprenorphine is poorly absorbed when swallowed.)

The reason for combining buprenorphine with naloxone is to prevent misuse. Naloxone is very poorly absorbed from under the tongue, through the cheek, or if swallowed. So the naloxone in the combination product is just a bystander if the combination is used as intended. If, however, the buprenorphine/naloxone combination medication is crushed, snorted, or injected, the naloxone acts to cut short or block the experience of a pleasurable feeling from the buprenorphine and to precipitate withdrawal.

Here's a case example: A patient experiencing a severe relapse had such desperate cravings for opioids that he melted down and injected his full dose of Suboxone®, which had been given to him to take under the tongue as part of opioid addiction treatment. He described the experience this way: "First, I felt the most unbelievable high but before I could count to 10, I experienced a sudden crash, with the worst withdrawal

I've had in a long time. I literally thought I was going to die on the spot."

What is naltrexone?

A third group of FDA-approved medications contain naltrexone, a long-acting medication similar to the reversal medication naloxone. Oral naltrexone lasts for a day, injectable depot naltrexone (known as Vivitrol®) lasts for a month, and some pharmacies are advertising additional forms that last 6 months or longer. (These very-long acting forms have not undergone a safety review by the FDA).

Because naltrexone serves as only a blocker on the opioid receptor, it can easily precipitate withdrawal in someone who has recently taken opioids. As a result, doctors should wait until a patient has not taken any opioids for 7 to 10 days before giving a dose of naltrexone. Since this period of abstinence can be quite difficult for someone with active opioid addiction to accomplish, naltrexone rarely is suitable for people who show up at an emergency department or an outpatient clinic seeking help. It is more appropriate for people who have experienced long periods of abstinence. For example, people leaving residential settings who do not want or cannot take methadone or buprenorphine may benefit from starting injectable naltrexone prior to discharge.

Clinical studies have shown that when people are able to take naltrexone, it works about as well as buprenorphine in suppressing illicit opioid use.[23] However, getting people to start naltrexone has been more difficult than getting individuals to start buprenorphine. In addition, for the injectable form of naltrexone, most people take only one or two doses and then stop. That may be a major reason why naltrexone treatment in practice has not been found to be as associated with the same reductions in overdoses as methadone and buprenorphine.[24] Researchers are actively looking at ways to speed up the process for getting patients safely started on injectable naltrexone.

Which is the best medication to take for opioid addiction?

There is no one-size-fits-all approach to treating opioid addiction. In considering which medication to use, several questions can help.

1. *How severe is the opioid addiction?* People with a severe condition—reflected in heavy use by injection that dominates their daily life—may experience greater benefit from methadone than the other two medications. Those who are not experiencing severe symptoms may do well on buprenorphine or injectable naltrexone.

2. *Which medication has the person tried in the past, and what happened?* Many people have tried at least one of the medications, either as part of treatment or on their own and can describe whether it helped them feel better, made them feel worse, or did not do much. A common story is that someone achieved remission and recovery with a particular medication but stopped taking it and relapsed. In such a case, this same medication is a good place to start. On the other hand, if the person never stabilized on an adequate trial of a particular medication, it's best to try something different.

3. *Are there other medical or social factors that favor one medication over the others?* Such factors include what types of other medical and psychiatric conditions the person may have, their social circumstances, and how closely the individual needs to be monitored taking the medication.

For example, relevant conditions include:

- *Pregnancy.* Injectable naltrexone currently is not recommended for pregnant women. Methadone and buprenorphine are the standards of care.
- *Severe heart and lung disease.* Because of the lower risk of sedation, buprenorphine may be better than methadone.

- *Heart rhythm problems.* Methadone can increase the risk for a heart arrhythmia called Torsade de Pointe. For this reason, people at higher risk for this problem may be better off with buprenorphine than methadone.
- *Abdominal problems.* Methadone can also cause more severe constipation than the other two medications, so may be best to avoid in people who have had extensive abdominal surgery or recurrent bowel obstruction.

Since it is simpler to switch from buprenorphine to methadone than the other way around, when it is a toss-up between the two medications, starting with buprenorphine often makes sense. It is possible to get a good sense of whether buprenorphine will work within about a month of treatment at appropriate doses.

Once a medication has been chosen, some thought should be given to the setting. Someone who has a significant history of selling illicit substances may do best in a supervised opioid treatment program. There, she can be monitored more closely to make sure she is taking her medication appropriately, compared to seeing a primary care physician for a prescription for buprenorphine once a week or once a month.

Informed by these and other considerations, the decision about which medication to take, if any, is best made jointly between the patient and healthcare provider. Ultimately, it is the patient who must take the medication and go through the process of change.

How long should I take a medication for opioid addiction?

For as long as needed. Unfortunately, some insurance companies and treatment programs set arbitrary limits, such as 3 or 6 months, on medication. Some peers and family members urge people to stop medications as soon as possible to achieve a "drug-free" recovery.

This is terrible advice. Recovery has to do with not misusing opioids, taking steps to put your life back together, and living a productive life with meaning and purpose. Medications help people focus on that process. In fact, stopping medication use is associated with a significant risk of relapse, in some studies between 50% to 80%.[25,26] With relapse comes a risk of fatal overdose. Pressuring someone to stop taking methadone, buprenorphine, or naltrexone makes about as much sense as pressuring someone with HIV to stop taking antiviral medication or asking someone with diabetes to stop taking insulin.

Some people choose to take medications for opioid addiction for the rest of their lives, which is an entirely reasonable decision. Others, on their own time, decide to taper off—which also can be a reasonable decision. One factor for individuals and their physicians to consider is that stopping treatment is associated with particularly high relapse rates during the first 3 to 5 years of recovery. Once a decision is made to lower the dose, it is important to take stock along the way of whether cravings are returning. This may signal a need to adjust the treatment medication dose and wait before proceeding further.

Does evidence support the use of marijuana as an effective treatment for opioid addiction?

No. In a comprehensive review, the National Academies of Science, Engineering, and Medicine found that "there is no or insufficient evidence to support or refute the conclusion that cannabis or cannabinoids are an effective treatment for . . . achieving abstinence in the use of addictive substances."[27]

Does evidence support the use of the botanical kratom as an effective treatment for opioid addiction?

No. Kratom, a botanical plant commonly found in southeast Asia, contains two opioid-like chemicals among many other components. People who chew the leaves or drink tea made from the plant report increased energy as well as sensations of pleasure. More recently, people have turned to kratom pills and capsules to reduce their use of prescription opioids or to "cure" opioid addiction. However, no studies have supported kratom's effectiveness as a treatment for opioid addiction. Moreover, according to the Mayo Clinic, "research suggests that [kratom] leads to more health problems than it solves."[28] FDA Commissioner Scott Gottlieb has stated, "Far from treating addiction, we've determined that kratom is an opioid analogue that may actually contribute to the opioid epidemic and puts patients at risk of serious side effects."[29] Reported adverse effects from kratom include nausea and vomiting, seizures, and hallucinations.

Does evidence support ibogaine as an effective treatment for opioid addiction?

No. Ibogaine is a hallucinogen derived from the root barks of the Iboga tree. Some have claimed that taking ibogaine has solved their opioid addiction after just a single dose; however, there have been no successful clinical trials of ibogaine for opioid addiction. There are, instead, 27 case reports of fatalities, most related to heart arrhythmias. In one review, researchers wrote, "With limited medical supervision, these are risky experiments and more ibogaine-related deaths are likely to occur, particularly in those with pre-existing cardiac conditions and those taking concurrent medications."[30]

How is pain managed in someone being treated for opioid addiction?

People in treatment for an opioid addiction often have pain. This pain may be short-term, as a result of injuries or surgeries, or long lasting. There is evidence that people with opioid addiction tend to have a higher sensitivity to pain, but it is not clear why. One possibility is that this sensitivity preceded (and perhaps contributed to) the opioid addiction. An alternative explanation is that prolonged opioid exposure "resets" the pain system. Regardless of the reason, it is important to attend to pain in patients with opioid addiction, as failure to do so increases the risk of relapse.

Many healthcare professionals and sometimes even patients erroneously think that the once-daily methadone or buprenorphine taken for opioid addiction is sufficient to treat pain. This is false for two reasons. The first reason has to do with frequency of dosing. To be optimally effective for pain, methadone, and buprenorphine must be taken 3, sometimes even 4, times a day. This frequency of dosing is recommended because the pain-relieving properties of these medications wear off after 6 to 8 hours. Taking a single dose once a day treats opioid addiction, not pain. Second, tolerance develops to the minimal pain relief provided by once a day dosing of methadone or buprenorphine. So patients cannot rely on their usual regimen for addiction treatment to control pain adequately.

It is optimal for pain in patients with opioid addiction to be controlled through a combination of physical therapy, acupuncture, other types of care, and non-opioid medications. In some cases, however, additional opioids may be required. When this happens, the treating physician may be able to split the dose of methadone or buprenorphine so that it is taken multiple times a day. There might also be a need to increase the dose temporarily to overcome the tolerance that the patient has developed over time. An alternative approach is to add a sufficient dose of a new opioid.

If someone in treatment for opioid addiction does need other opioids for pain, a few strategies can help reduce the risk for misuse or relapse. First, the patient should enlist a trusted family member to help monitor the medications. This helps maintain trust with the family member and facilitates early identification of problems, should they occur. Second, the patient should stop taking the opioid pain medications if familiar symptoms of cravings or euphoria develop. Third, the patient should ask the prescriber to write for the smallest number of tablets necessary given the clinical need. Finally, the patient should let the addiction treatment provider know which medications were prescribed. This will help if a drug test un-expectedly comes back positive for the pain medication.

Some people in recovery elect not to take additional opioids for pain, fearful that it will negatively impact their recovery. [31] Such a choice is their right. In such a case, the provider should develop an alternative plan, rather than ignore the presence of pain.

What is "detox"?

"Detox" is not addiction treatment. Detox refers to the process of easing the withdrawal symptoms from opioids by providing medical care for a period that usually lasts from 3 to 7 days.

Detox is not necessary. The effective medications metha-done or buprenorphine actually treat withdrawal. People do not need to go through detox to start ongoing therapy with these medications.

When utilized, detox may involve a few doses of methadone or buprenorphine in rapidly decreasing amounts, combined with other medications to address specific withdrawal symptoms. Or it may just involve these other medications alone, particularly if the person's goal is to start injectable depot naltrexone. For example, the medication clonidine treats the el-evated blood pressure and heart rate seen with withdrawal; ibuprofen addresses joint and muscle aches; dicyclomine, ab-dominal cramps; loperamide, diarrhea; and trazodone, sleep-lessness. The FDA recently approved a new medicine called Lucemyra™, otherwise known as lofexidine, to help treat the symptoms of opioid withdrawal.[32] Lofexidine is similar to clonidine and has been used in Europe for the treatment of high blood pressure and opioid withdrawal for decades.

Detox should not even be called "detox." A better term is withdrawal management. Even with the best protocol and multiple medications, withdrawal management can often be stressful and uncomfortable for patients. The biggest problem with withdrawal management, however, is the high relapse risk following its completion. To reduce this danger, it is important to follow up with effective treatment for the underlying addiction as soon as possible.

What is the role of counseling and other mental health care in the treatment of opioid addiction?

A critical role for counseling in the treatment of opioid addiction is education. Patients often do not understand addiction. Counseling helps people appreciate the nature of addiction and its consequences, the importance of triggers for drug use, and healthy approaches for managing symptoms in the short and long term. This type of education is often done in groups with information that can then be reinforced through individual sessions.

Another important role of counseling is retraining the brain. Often, people are not aware of their own triggers for opioid misuse. Through counseling, patients identify these cues and develop healthy coping strategies. Counseling also helps people to assess why these strategies sometimes fail and to develop more effective responses. This process helps uncouple cravings from actual use.

There are different types of counseling approaches. Two of the most common are:

- *Cognitive-behavioral therapy.* This approach helps people develop specific mental techniques for coping with triggers. This therapy often takes time as patients practice and modify these techniques. Cognitive-behavioral therapy does not work for everyone, however. For example, it may be less effective for people with untreated mental illness or significant traumatic brain injury.
- *Motivational interviewing.* With motivational interviewing, through a series of steps, the health professional works

with the patient to set self-determined goals, connect dots between behaviors and their consequences, increase motivation to make changes, and support changes once they have been made. Some experts have likened motivational interviewing to a dance between the professional and the patient as successful outcomes depend on collaboration, negotiation, and a partnership—rather than the professional telling the patient what to do without regard for whether the person actually wants to follow through.

These two counseling techniques have broad applicability beyond opioid addiction. As a result, they can be incorporated into different types of medical settings. It may sometimes seem that counseling can only be delivered by trained addiction counselors. In fact, primary care physicians can use these approaches to counsel their patients on how to manage their diabetes and their high blood pressure, as well as their opioid addiction, as part of a visit that also involves the patient getting a buprenorphine prescription or an injection of depot naltrexone.

Counseling can also highlight the need for additional mental healthcare. It is important for people receiving addiction treatment to be assessed for untreated mental illness, particularly depression, post-traumatic stress symptoms, and bipolar disease. Effective care for these and other psychiatric conditions can substantially increase the odds of success in addiction treatment and greatly improve quality of life.

What is the role of peers in the treatment of opioid addiction?

It is becoming increasingly common to find peers in recovery from addiction working in different clinical settings—from emergency departments to addiction treatment centers. Their title is often "peer recovery specialist." The rationale for this position is that peers with lived experience of addiction can understand, relate to, and better engage with others who are facing similar struggles. As part of their training, peers may be required to obtain a certification demonstrating competencies in such areas as ethics and the basics of addiction.

Peer recovery specialists are not clinicians. This means their roles in clinical settings center around providing resources, assisting with case management and linkage to different treatment and recovery support services, and providing emotional support.

What is the role of a residential (inpatient) setting in the treatment of opioid addiction?

Most people with opioid addiction do well in community-based treatment programs. Residential care for persons with opioid addiction is recommended in a few specific situations. For example, when someone also suffers from significant addiction to benzodiazepines or alcohol, a medically monitored environment minimizes the risk of withdrawal seizures from these other substances. If a person is having difficulty stabilizing their opioid addiction in an outpatient setting despite an adequate dose of an effective treatment medication and intensive counseling, a brief residential stay may be helpful.

Despite a relatively limited need for residential treatment, many people demand it. Public officials promise greater access to "beds," insurers are pressed to cover this care, and millions of capital dollars are devoted to building new facilities. This drive reflects, in part, the compelling personal testimony that some graduates of residential treatment programs are able to provide. It also reflects the intuition that many people have that a change of environment is therapeutic.

A new location and a quiet place to recuperate may indeed help some people achieve a remission from opioid addiction. For many others, however, removal from the community for 30 or 90 days or even 180 days makes it more difficult to learn how to cope with the stressors of daily life. Many strategies developed in residential treatment fall apart as soon as people are exposed to their regular reminders of use. Making matters worse, few residential treatment programs offer access to medications for treatment, and fewer still are able to establish strong aftercare programs that assure ongoing care and supports.

Which patients would stand to benefit from residential treatment is a matter of clinical judgment (aided by professional guidance and thorough patient assessments) and patient preference. At a minimum, residential treatment programs should offer access to all 3 FDA-approved medications, link patients directly to follow-up care, and closely monitor their outcomes.

What is the role of drug testing in the treatment of opioid addiction?

Drug testing can confirm progress in treatment and can identify lapses as early as possible so appropriate interventions can be provided. Testing is most commonly performed on urine samples and less commonly on special swabs that soak up saliva in the mouth. Because of cost and the time it takes to receive results, as well as questions about accuracy, hair testing is rarely used as part of addiction treatment.

Drug testing can reveal whether individuals have consumed certain opioids. However, testing does not provide information about the manner in which opioids were consumed. Nor does testing reveal how much was consumed.

Most opioids or their byproducts stay in the body for 3 to 4 days, so a drug test will reflect use during that time. Testing more frequently than once a week generally does not make sense, because repeated positives could all be due to the same episode of use.

A commonly used drug test assesses for the presence or absence of opiates as a class. This test turns positive in the presence of those opioids that are derived directly from poppy plants, including morphine and codeine. It also turns positive in the presence of several specific opioids with similar chemical structures, including hydromorphone and hydrocodone.

A positive result could even be due to heroin, because heroin is rapidly metabolized in the body to morphine. If the opiate test is particularly sensitive, a positive result could even be due to eating poppy seeds, which contain a minuscule amount of opium. This test is often used when people start treatment and at regular intervals throughout treatment, with a frequency that depends on how people are doing. (Neither methadone nor buprenorphine cause a positive result on this test.)

Other tests assess specifically for the presence (or absence) of specific opioids, such as oxycodone, oxymorphone, buprenorphine, methadone, fentanyl, and tramadol. Many of these tests require more sophisticated (and expensive) testing equipment. Some laboratories provide information on the specific levels of opioids in the urine. However, because there are so many variables that affect the level of a substance within someone's bodily fluids, these numbers are typically meaningless by themselves. The more specific tests are used when it is important to understand exactly which opioid someone has used.

Here's a case example. A 58-year-old man in treatment with methadone provides a urine sample every month, which is tested both for the presence of methadone and for the presence of opiates. One month, his tests are positive for methadone, as expected, but also for opiates, which is unexpected. His doctor is concerned that he may have relapsed to heroin. She calls the lab to ask them to run a more sophisticated test to figure out what caused the opiate positive result. A few days later, she gets the answer: codeine. When she talks with the patient, he admits to taking a pill from his wife that contained codeine. He agrees that he will leave his wife's pills alone in the future.

Healthcare providers should handle drug test results like they handle other laboratory test results: carefully. They should interpret the results in the context of the patient's clinical presentation, understand what might cause false-positive or false-negative results, and review the result and the interpretation with the patient. If there is no clear explanation for the test result or the patient disputes the clinician's interpretation, the provider should repeat the test or order a more sophisticated test to clarify the initial test result. Guidelines, such as from the American Society of Addiction Medicine, caution against providers making drastic treatment changes based on one drug test result.[33]

What is the role of my primary care provider in the treatment of opioid addiction?

As addiction treatment becomes more and more integrated with the rest of healthcare, expectations for primary care providers can, and should, grow. That's why you should expect your primary care provider to ask you clear, non-judgmental screening questions about the use and misuse of substances, including nicotine, alcohol, opioids, and other drugs. (Only with honest answers to these questions can the provider help you if there is a problem.)

If you acknowledge or the provider makes a diagnosis of an opioid use disorder, a few things should happen. First, the provider should ensure that you and your family have naloxone and know when and how to use it. Second, the provider should assess the severity of the condition and discuss effective treatment options. A growing number of primary care physicians, nurse practitioners, and physicians assistants can prescribe buprenorphine or injectable naltrexone to patients with opioid addiction within the primary care setting. Third, your primary care provider should continue to check in with you on how your recovery is going even years and decades later, just like they would check up on your diabetes or cancer when these are in remission.

If the primary care provider is not able to treat your opioid addiction in the office, he or she should work with you and your family to arrange treatment with a specialty addiction treatment provider.

Unfortunately, there are still too many primary care providers who either do not know about the different resources in their communities or do not want to get involved with their patients' addiction. Often, this is out of fear, bias, ignorance, or a belief that addiction is not a disease. Whatever the case, if a primary care provider is unwilling or unable to help with an opioid addiction, it may be time to switch to one who can.

What should I expect from my specialty addiction treatment provider?

Specialty addiction treatment providers can be physicians, nurse practitioners, physicians assistants, clinical social workers, professional counselors, or other healthcare professionals. Often, having a team of professionals with different clinical training and credentials is helpful in getting all your needs addressed. No matter their background, every professional should treat you with respect and provide clear, evidence-based information about different treatment options, including medications. Having physicians, nurse practitioners, or physician assistants as part of the team is important because only they can prescribe and adjust medications for opioid addiction.

Specialty addiction providers should also know their limits. If you have questions they cannot answer or need different care from what their program offers, they should refer you elsewhere.

When people with opioid addiction seek care, they are often feeling desperate, emotionally and physically in distress, and ambivalent about long-term recovery. They may have experienced a significant amount of trauma either prior to developing their addiction or as part of active use. Specialty addiction treatment providers should be aware of best practices in trauma-informed care so they can effectively engage with and treat patients—and not retraumatize them.

Specialty addiction treatment providers should make sure you are connected to and coordinate care with other healthcare providers so everyone is clear on the treatments being provided. They may also be able to treat you directly for certain health conditions, including hepatitis C or depression.

What should I expect from other clinicians in the healthcare system?

Given the scale of the opioid epidemic, every healthcare provider caring for patients should be prepared to refer to effective addiction treatment. No professional should react to people in need with anger, stigma, or discrimination. And many clinicians—including emergency department physicians, hospitalists, and specialists who provide ongoing care for their patients—should be prepared to start treatment with effective medications.

What confidentiality protections exist for treatment for opioid addiction?

The Health Insurance and Portability Accountability Act, otherwise known as HIPAA, is the law that protects the privacy of all patient specific health information. This law generally allows the sharing of health information with all clinicians taking care of a patient. The privacy of addiction treatment information is further protected by a federal regulation called CFR 42 Part 2. This federal law prohibits the sharing of information about addiction treatment with anyone, even other clinicians, without the specific written consent of the patient. There are a handful of exceptions, including severe medical emergencies and threats by patients to hurt themselves or others.

The federal government created CFR 42 Part 2 in the 1970s to encourage people to seek treatment for addiction without fear that their confidential information would be used against them by law enforcement and the criminal justice system. Much has changed since then with respect to medical records, information sharing, and the approach to addiction treatment.

There is now growing interest in changing CFR 42 Part 2 to make its protections align more with HIPAA. The goal of such changes is to improve health information sharing between treating providers. Many people believe that this will further the integration of addiction treatment into medical practice and reduce stigma. However, the underlying goal of the regulation—to keep information from leading to violations of privacy or the prosecution of patients—remains important.

7

OPIOIDS AND PREGNANCY

What are the risks of opioid exposure during pregnancy?

Opioids cross the placenta. That means when a pregnant woman consumes opioids, some pass through to her developing fetus.

The most direct impact of opioids on the fetus is the development of tolerance. Just as the mother's body becomes accustomed to a regular dose of opioids, so does that of the fetus. If the mother goes into withdrawal prior to delivery, so does the fetus. This can create distress in the womb and even fetal death.

There are indirect impacts, too. Women who snort or inject opioids are at risk for becoming infected with HIV, the hepatitis C virus, and certain bacteria. These pathogens can cross the placenta, and when they do, they can infect the developing fetus. In rare cases, pregnant women develop heart valve infections from drug use, and infectious material can break off and infect the placenta. This can trigger a life-threatening infection for both the mother and the fetus.

The most serious threat to the developing fetus is the risk of overdose in the pregnant woman. A growing fetus is dependent on oxygen and other nutrients from the mother's blood supply. When a pregnant woman overdoses, even if it is not fatal to her, the developing fetus may suffer profound effects, even death.

These facts underscore the importance of providing effective treatment to pregnant women with addiction.

How is opioid addiction treated during pregnancy?

The standard of care for pregnant women with opioid addiction includes treatment with either methadone or buprenorphine.[1] This standard exists for three reasons.

First, it is possible for women to start these treatments, which are both opioid medications, without experiencing significant withdrawal, which could be harmful to the fetus.

Second, both medications are highly effective. Pregnant women who receive them commonly stop using illicit opioids. This both lowers their risk of overdose and creates the opportunity to focus on their own health and the health of their future child. That's why experts advise against withdrawal management, even if medically monitored.[2]

Third, women greatly benefit from support and services available in treatment programs, both before and after delivery. The stress of becoming a new mom can lead to relapse, so these extra supports, in addition to the medication, can help keep moms on track in recovery.

Which medication is most effective for pregnant women with opioid addiction?

Methadone and buprenorphine are both good options for pregnant women with opioid addiction. Both medications work similarly to reduce relapse and stabilize addiction.

In clinical studies comparing the two medications, pregnant women stayed in treatment slightly longer with methadone compared to buprenorphine.

Because pregnancy alters the way a woman's body handles some medications, doctors may need to adjust the dose of methadone during and after pregnancy. For women who were taking methadone before becoming pregnant, the dose may need to be increased during pregnancy to maintain effectiveness, and then reduced after delivery to avoid excessive fatigue and sleepiness. The need for dose changes does not seem to occur as much with buprenorphine. In studies, infants born to women taking buprenorphine spent a couple of fewer days in the hospital before going home and needed less medicine after birth compared to the infants born to mothers taking methadone.[3] Ultimately, the choice of medication should be a decision between the woman and her healthcare provider.

What is neonatal abstinence syndrome?

Neonatal abstinence syndrome—otherwise known as NAS—describes the symptoms newborn babies often experience when born to a mother who has taken opioids during her pregnancy. Essentially, NAS is opioid withdrawal, as experienced by the baby. As a result of the opioid epidemic, rates of NAS have grown to more than 30 per 1,000 in some states.[4]

Not every baby born to a woman taking an opioid during pregnancy will develop NAS. Between 40% and 80% of pregnant women using heroin will have babies with NAS, while only 5% to 20% of women taking a prescription opioid medication do so.[5] As with all opioids, the treatment medications methadone and buprenorphine can cause NAS.

Other factors influence the development of NAS. Babies born to women who also use cocaine, take alprazolam (Xanax®) or other benzodiazepines, smoke cigarettes, or drink alcohol have a higher risk for NAS compared to women who only use opioids. Recently, scientists have discovered several genetic variants in the opioid receptors of newborns that may increase their risk for developing NAS.[6]

Untreated, a baby with NAS will have symptoms that include sustained crying, difficulty soothing, tremors, poor feeding, vomiting, diarrhea, and difficulty sleeping for a period of days to weeks. A small percentage of newborns with NAS have seizures. The good news is that NAS is treatable.

How is neonatal abstinence syndrome treated?

Treatment for neonatal abstinence syndrome, or NAS, involves both medication and a supportive environment.

The most commonly used medication for NAS is morphine, in very small doses. The treating clinician finds a sufficient dose to control the symptoms and then lowers the dose over time until the medication is not needed at all. More recently, studies suggest that using small doses of methadone or buprenorphine may lead to better outcomes than morphine treatment.[7,8]

In addition to medication, hospitals should establish a supportive environment for babies with NAS. To support bonding between mother and baby, hospitals should allow rooming-in for the baby and the mother, rather than having the baby separated from the mother in the intensive care unit. Other recommended practices include swaddling and breastfeeding. Even mothers who are receiving treatment with methadone or buprenorphine can breastfeed, because so little of the medication passes into breast milk. Some hospitals add dim lighting, soft music, and special efforts to reduce extraneous noise and provide a calm environment for mother and baby.

Some hospitals are adopting a new approach to NAS that involves more rapid reductions in the dose of morphine.[9] Proponents have claimed that a rapid taper is safe and less costly to the healthcare system. However, some experts have expressed concern that this new approach does not pay enough attention to signs of distress in newborns. The National Institutes of Health has recently prioritized studying the best approaches for the treatment of NAS.

Is a baby with neonatal abstinence syndrome "born addicted"?

No. Babies with NAS are experiencing a withdrawal syndrome, but withdrawal is not the same as addiction. Addiction is characterized by pathological craving and compulsion that drives someone to keep using a substance even in the face of severe negative consequences to the person's life, including the threat of death. Babies are not capable of having addiction.

What are the long-term effects of opioid use during pregnancy?

There is a tendency for people to panic about drug use by pregnant women.[10] Three decades ago, sensational magazine stories fueled fear of an epidemic of "crack babies." A July 1986 *Newsweek* article called newborns of addicted mothers "heirs of America's deadly romance with cocaine"[11] and noted "doctors can only guess at the scope" of the problems the children would have. A September 1988 *TIME* article, titled "Crack Comes to the Nursery," reported:

> Even one "hit" of crack can irreparably damage a fetus or breast-fed baby. At birth the babies display obvious signs of crack exposure—tremors, irritability and lethargy—that may belie the seriousness of the harm done. These symptoms may disappear in a week or more, but the underlying damage remains.[12]

Central to the concept of babies harmed by crack exposure in utero was the profound distance between a mother and her child. The former was seen as the perpetrator; the latter, as the victim. During the 1980s, many poor women were prosecuted for crack use during pregnancy.[13]

In fact, both mom and baby were suffering together. Subsequent studies of prenatal cocaine exposure showed no major effect on long-term developmental outcome[14]; the greater culprit in poor development and health was identified as poverty.[15] Misguided panic over such infants obscured the single most important intervention for the future of the baby—helping her mother succeed in life.

So it is with opioid exposure as well. There is no shortage of reporters focusing on the "heartbreaking development"[16] of an increase in the number of newborns affected by their mothers' opioid use; one article, titled "Drug Addicts at Birth,"[17] led with a district attorney's concern over the "innocent victims." Only the rare journalist recognizes that, although newborns may display symptoms of withdrawal, they are not addicted. Fewer still write about the critical importance of addressing difficult social circumstances on the developing child.

Studies on the impact of opioids on developing brains are difficult to conduct. That's because it is challenging to tease out the effects of the opioids themselves from the effects of everything that comes with them—other drugs, social instability at home, exposure to violence, and poverty. So researchers have found mixed results, with some evidence for an increased risk of behavioral disorders and lower test scores years later.[18] At the same time, it is clear that exposure is not destiny, and many children are able to do quite well.

Compared to the unclear impact of exposure to opioids on the developing brain, it is well established that adverse social circumstances pose very serious risks to developing children. Unstable and dangerous home environments are associated with a broad range of subsequent effects, including problems in school, mental health problems, physical disorders such as obesity and diabetes, and subsequent addiction.[19]

To prevent these problems, pregnant women should be encouraged to receive treatment with methadone and buprenorphine, even though these medications can cause NAS. By treating the mother's addiction, these medications stabilize the home environment and put the family in the best position to succeed.

For their part, babies should receive treatment for NAS with small and decreasing amounts of opioids, as this reduces distressing symptoms and makes it easier for parents to care for the child. Studies have found that treatment of NAS with opioids does not pose any additional risk to babies' development.[20]

More broadly, those concerned about the long-term effects of opioid exposure should support providing a broad set of services to women with a recent history of addiction—including before, during, and after pregnancy. There are a number of model programs for new families that include such components as home visiting from nurses, free diapers, and free books.[21] Scaling up these programs is likely to help many opioid-exposed children thrive.

Should women who use opioids breastfeed?

It depends. Breastfeeding is encouraged for women who received adequate prenatal care and are not using illicit opioids or other illicit drugs. Women receiving methadone or buprenorphine for addiction treatment can breastfeed too, because these medications are present in breastmilk in insignificant amounts.

Breastfeeding is discouraged for women who can pass infectious diseases (such as HIV) to their newborns, women who are taking other medications that do pass into the breastmilk (such as some anti-seizure medications), and women who are continuing to use illicit substances, including marijuana. Women who use opioids should discuss breastfeeding with a healthcare provider.

8

OPIOIDS AND TEENAGERS

How has the opioid epidemic in the United States affected teenagers?

From 1991 to 2012, the misuse of opioid prescription medications among teenagers more than doubled.[1] So did the rate of opioid addiction,[2] the rate of hospitalizations for overdose,[3] and the rate of fatal overdose.[4] In 2014, close to 500,000 US youth between the ages of 12 and 17 reported misuse of opioid pills, with more than 150,000 reporting the symptoms of opioid addiction.[5]

What are the characteristics of opioid addiction among teenagers?

Opioid addiction often starts with misusing prescription medications, most often obtained from friends and family. Only 1 in 5 teenagers start using opioids as a result of a prescription from their physician.[6]

Teenagers often believe, falsely, that prescription opioids are not addictive. As their use increases, however, teenagers might start hanging out with a different crowd, withdraw from their usual activities, or display symptoms such as depression, irritability, and anger. Teenagers may start showing significant impairment in school, have problems getting home on time, or experience trouble with the law. Opioid misuse often comes to light in the setting of an arrest—or an overdose.[7]

Opioid addiction in teenagers is very dangerous. In addition to the risk of overdose, teenagers may engage in risky sex, use other dangerous drugs like cocaine and methamphetamines, and attempt suicide.[8] Heroin use appears to be associated with the highest levels of risky behaviors.[9]

Here's a case example: A 16-year old girl smokes cigarettes, uses marijuana, and experiments with other drugs with her friends. When opioid pills are added to the mix, she experiences a special euphoria and wants more. She starts taking pills from her own family and stealing from the medicine cabinets of her neighbors. She finds she needs more opioids to achieve the same effect, and experiences withdrawal symptoms when she does not have access to opioids for more than a few days. She starts to lie to her parents and ignore her schoolwork and other activities. She begins to crush and snort the pills for a more intense high, and steals money to purchase opioids on the street. Her parents figure out the problem only after they find her unresponsive and call 911.

Is treatment effective for teenagers with opioid addiction?

Yes. As for adults, there is effective and life-saving treatment for opioid addiction for teenagers. A major challenge, however, is that fewer than 1 in 20 teenagers with a problem recognizes the need for help.[10] Parents and guardians have a vital role to play in identifying opioid misuse and helping teenagers reach care.

A common first stop is residential treatment. Inpatient care or a residential treatment program that includes close medical monitoring is necessary for adolescents with extensive use of other dangerous substances, including alcohol and benzodiazepines (such as Xanax®). This is because withdrawal from these substances can be life-threatening.

A short period in residential treatment can also be helpful to youth when the home situation is unstable. There is evidence that a cooling off period for the teenager, as well as for parents and siblings, can help with the development of new coping skills before another try at home.[11]

For those teenagers who go into residential treatment, ongoing care after discharge is critical. Peer groups, counseling, and treatment of other medical and psychiatric disorders can help teenagers stay stable, continue their education, and begin the process of recovery.

Whether or not treatment starts in a residential setting, there is solid evidence that medication treatment helps teenagers with opioid addiction. Researchers have found that buprenorphine helps teenagers stay in treatment, reduces their misuse of opioids, lowers their chance of obtaining HIV and hepatitis C, and promotes long-term recovery.[12,13] Yet many addiction counselors advise families not to use medications, and only a minority of treatment programs even offer medications to adolescents with opioid addiction.[14]

An important element of treatment of adolescents is support for the family. Family therapy is recommended to identify points of conflict and develop shared ways to resolve them. Families should also try to break out of the isolation and shame that can set in with a struggling teen at home. Parents and siblings can benefit from joining non-judgmental support groups and may also need care for their own medical and psychiatric conditions.

Extended family and friends have a vital role to play. They can help by providing respite for primary caregivers as well as by developing special projects and activities with teenagers and their siblings.

Should parents of teenagers who use opioids keep naloxone in the home?

Yes. As a precaution, parents should have naloxone at home to use in case of an overdose. Parents should also be trained in how to administer this life-saving medication. The easiest way to obtain naloxone is to talk to your local pharmacist. In many places, there is a standing order for naloxone, meaning that anyone can get a dose.[15] If this is not the case in your area, your pharmacist may direct you to your doctor or to public health agencies that may be holding trainings and distributing doses directly.

What should parents do in a crisis?

There are moments when teenagers take actions that put their own lives, and the lives of others, at risk. Options for parents include:

- *Call crisis services.* Some areas of the country offer specialized mental health and addiction teams that make house calls. These teams include professionals who are trained to diffuse tension, provide services on site, and make plans for follow-up treatment and care. Parents and guardians should find out if there is a respected crisis service program in the area and keep the number handy. In addition to house calls, crisis services may offer drop-in programs in the area.
- *Take the teenager to the emergency department.* When youth are a risk to themselves or others, or fundamentally out of control, the emergency department can assess for any medical problems and consider whether a psychiatric hospitalization is appropriate.
- *Call 911.* In the event of imminent danger that is not able to be addressed by another means, there is no substitute for calling 911. If successful, first responders can protect the youth and those around him or her. Often, the call will lead to a transport to the emergency department. However, there are also risks to this approach. Untrained first responders can escalate the danger, not reduce it. It is very important for those who call 911 to explain the medical history of the youth so that responders can be

prepared and, ideally, a team trained for these types of emergencies can be deployed.

Are there scams targeting parents of teenagers with addiction?

Yes. "Frustrated, exhausted and frightened parents who contact troubled teen programs—often at a time of crisis—may be vulnerable to salespeople who hustle them into expensive contracts," explains a website devoted to the "safe, therapeutic, and appropriate use of residential treatment." It continues: "Please slow down."[16]

This is good advice. There are hundreds of risky programs advertising to parents worried about their teenagers' drug use. Some of these programs are entirely unregulated. Others may hold licenses or accreditation but do not deserve them. Some offer brutal "wilderness" activities, like long hikes under the baking sun. Others feature "scared straight" programs, which may have kids sleep in coffins or spend nights in a jail cell.

A report from the Government Accountability Office found that in one year alone, more than 1,500 staff members in residential programs in 33 states were "involved in incidents of abuse."[17] The report found "untrained staff," "lack of adequate nourishment," and "reckless or negligent operating practices" as common factors in 10 deaths of teenagers in these programs. One mother of a child who died said:

> I understood there would be highly trained and qualified people with [my daughter] who could handle any emergency . . . they boasted of a 13-year flawless safety record, [and] I thought to myself "why should I worry? Why would anything happen to her?"[18]

Three days into the program, her daughter died of heatstroke while hiking after "forced march, night hikes, and limited food and water."[19]

In 2014, CNN reported on a Colorado program for teens with addiction that was sued 15 times for "verbal and sexual abuse, unauthorized discontinuance of psychotropic medication, and fraud." The report asked, "How did an unlicensed professional, who led people to believe he was a medical doctor, run a facility for adolescents with mental illness and drug abuse problems for decades, despite complaint after complaint to state regulators alleging abuse?"[20]

Again and again, worried parents spend thousands of dollars, or even tens of thousands of dollars, on programs that are more likely to make matters worse than help their teenagers. Fraud is so common that the Federal Trade Commission has posted a website devoted to protecting consumers.[21] Parents should never agree to a program based on a high-pressure phone call. The agency also recommends that parents considering residential treatment for their teenagers take a number of steps, including "ask questions, ask for proof or support for claims about staff credentials, program accreditation, and endorsements," visit the program, and "get all policies and promises in writing."[22]

9

OPIOIDS AND FAMILIES

What do I do if I suspect my family member is misusing opioids?

Family members are often the first to notice that there is something amiss with their loved ones. Parents might notice that their teenager is becoming more sullen or non-communicative than usual, or grandparents might notice that opioid medications go missing after their adult grandchild has been to visit. When family members suspect that their loved one may be misusing opioids, whether prescribed or not, there are a few things to do.

- Try not to become overly anxious. That is difficult to do as the natural tendency is to react with fear, anxiety, shame, disappointment, and anger. Remind yourself that addiction is a disease, not a moral failing or lack of will-power, and that your loved one may be feeling many of the same emotions you are.
- Talk with your loved one about your concern, using a non-judgmental and caring approach, language, posture, and tone of voice. Even with this approach, your loved one may become defensive. Do not take this personally.
- Let your loved one know that you want to help, that you care for his or her safety and well-being, and that you are not judging him or her.

- Make sure you have naloxone easily accessible in the house, should it be needed.
- Share your concerns with your loved one's doctor, ideally with your loved one present.
- Seek assistance for yourself and your other family members as these situations often evoke different reactions in different people; just like the person potentially misusing opioids needs support, so does the rest of the family.
- Remember that people with hazardous opioid use or opioid addiction may not be able to see the problem they have. You can help them connect the dots in their behavior by discussing the behaviors and consequences and by not impugning their character.
- Connect your loved one with effective treatment.

How can I help connect my family member with opioid addiction to effective treatment?

Because finding effective treatment can seem difficult or even overwhelming, it is helpful to break the process down into a few specific steps.

Step 1: Call a trusted clinician to provide care or referral

Ideally, your family member already has a primary care doctor or perhaps even a psychiatrist. If not, call your own. Local clinicians should have a good sense of where to start. The best option may be a local clinic or outpatient treatment program, where patients can receive high-quality care while working on a variety of critical issues that affect their daily lives. If your doctor is unable to help, proceed to Step 2.

Step 2: Contact a state or local health department

Health departments often provide directories of or connections to effective treatment services. Some even host or operate telephone crisis lines that can get people connected to care. If no success, try Step 3.

Step 3: Call the federal hotline

The Substance Abuse and Mental Health Services Administration maintains an online list of treatment providers, including providers who hold the special license to prescribe buprenorphine. The 24-hour number is 1-800-662-HELP (4357).

How can I tell if a treatment program is high quality?

Even when a program comes highly recommended, family members of individuals with opioid addiction should assess the situation for themselves. Six key questions to ask before starting treatment are:

Who Is providing the care?

Among the professionals, there should be a physician, nurse practitioner, or physician assistant who has the requisite knowledge, training, and credentials to provide or refer for treatment with buprenorphine, depot naltrexone, and methadone. This medical professional should be one of the first staff your loved one sees, preferably within a few hours of presenting for care. Other staff should include a licensed or certified addiction counselor or more advanced therapist. If these staff are in training, they should have a clinical supervisor who oversees everything they do and who you can contact. If a psychiatrist is not on staff, make sure a referral can be made to one if needed.

Is the program licensed and accredited and, if so, by whom?

Licensure and accreditation is a sign that the program is being held to specific standards. If those standards are not met, family members can contact state licensing and national accrediting organizations, such as the Joint Commission or

Commission on Accreditation of Rehabilitation Facilities, to voice their concerns.

What is the program's approach?

If the answer is "It's our special secret," "We rely on prayer alone," "Tough love," or anything else that does not seem to be based on science, be very skeptical. People can be harmed by these approaches.[1,2,3] Consider looking elsewhere or talking it over with a trusted clinician in your own community.

How are people with addiction treated?

Patients should be treated with respect and dignity, meaning they are made to feel welcome, comfortable, and attended to in a timely manner.

What happens if the patient is struggling or not responding to the initial therapy?

The answer should neither be "We discharge the person" nor "We call the authorities." Rather, the specialist or program should change the treatment plan. This may include referrals to other agencies that provide more intensive services than what the center itself can offer.

How does the treatment provider engage the family?

With the consent of an adult patient, family members should be able to receive updates and provide input to the treatment team. Even if an adult patient does not want their information shared, it is still possible for the treatment provider to listen to the family member, thank them for the information, and explain in general terms what treatment approaches are recommended for different clinical situations.

How can my family avoid residential treatment program scams?

People struggling with addiction and their families are vulnerable, often not knowing where to turn for effective care or ashamed to ask for help. This makes them marks for unscrupulous persons and businesses. The scams include so-called patient-brokers who promote toll-free numbers where people can call to get connected to treatment. These patient-brokers may offer free airfare to a residential treatment facility in beautiful locations like Florida or southern California, pick the person up at a designation of his or her choosing, and assist him or her in getting to the treatment facility.

What could possibly go wrong? A lot.

Once at the treatment facility, the patient's insurance or family member may be charged outrageous amounts for services that often amount to nothing more than a hotel room with spa-like activities—either until the insurance runs out or the family can no longer pay. Then the patient may be summarily discharged having received relatively little in the way of effective treatment and possibly at greater risk for overdose than when he or she came in.

The best way to avoid these scams is never to call advertised 1-800 numbers and instead to search for care through trusted clinicians, state and local health departments, and federal agencies. Particular skepticism is appropriate for any program that seems more like a vacation getaway than a healthcare facility.

Even when a residential treatment program does not seem like a scam, family members should ask tough questions before sending their loved one for care, including the following.

Does the residential treatment facility offer medications for addiction treatment?

Methadone, buprenorphine, and depot naltrexone help patients avoid illicit opioids and increase the chance of a remission and successful recovery. Treatment centers that put restrictions on which medication a patient can take or the dose or duration of any of these medications are not putting their patients in the best position to succeed. In some cases, they may be leaving people to suffer during the treatment stay and vulnerable to relapse and overdose upon discharge.

What is the nurse staffing?

Nurses should be available around the clock for patients being treated for opioid, alcohol, or sedative withdrawal. These patients need vital signs checked, withdrawal symptoms assessed, and medications administered to reduce the risk of dehydration, seizures, or the person leaving the facility prematurely.

What happens after the program ends?

If the answer is "We leave that up to the person or the family," look elsewhere. Residential treatment is typically shorter-term, acute care to stabilize the person but is not sufficient to help the individual sustain recovery. Residential facilities should work with the patient to develop an ongoing care and recovery plan, including identifying specific details about the who, what, when, and where of community-based services that address all the specific needs of the individual. One of these items should include a concrete plan for how patients will continue to receive any medication they may have started in the residential setting.

A visit to the residential facility can provide critical information about the care provided there. Family members should notice whether staff speak directly to the person with addiction, as well as to family members. Their language should be caring and without judgment. There should be a clear explanation of treatment expectation and outcomes. And the environment itself should be welcoming and clean, with private areas for clinical assessment, soap and hand sanitizer to minimize infection, and safe and clean quarters for sleeping.

It is common, especially for expensive residential treatment, for family members to ask about the success of the program—either through statistics or by seeking to speak with successful graduates. Be forewarned, however, that many residential programs provide unverifiable statistics. Also keep in mind that quality is not demonstrated by a few successful cases, however compelling. If a program seems too good to be true, it probably is.

What is "enabling"?

"Enabling" is a charged term. It is used to suggest that providing support to family members or loved ones with addiction may be counterproductive. "Enabling" suggests that providing transportation or housing or even affection to someone with an addiction might allow the person with the disease to simply continue using without consequences. Enabling is proscribed by a "tough love" philosophy that instructs family members and friends to believe that the more difficult life gets for someone with an addiction, the more likely it is for he or she to stop using drugs.

This philosophy, unfortunately, can backfire. People with an addiction generally respond well to consistent, clear, and non judgmental emotional support. That's why some effective treatment programs tell their new staff, "People with addiction have to see that you care before they care what you think." Empathy and understanding builds connections with people who often have suffered significant trauma in their lives; these connections are vital to the process of recovery. This is as true for family and friends as it is for treatment providers. People with addiction will seek help from those they trust. Rather than "enabling" an addiction, engagement and support can help build the foundation for health.

At the same time, families need not provide individuals who have an active addiction with money or housing or tolerate theft or physical threats. When spending time with or sharing living space with a loved one with addiction, family and friends should set and implement clear parameters for appropriate behavior. Together with the affected person, families should establish plans for what happens if established expectations of behavior are not met. These discussions should take place in the context of "We're here for you when you need help with your health," rather than "Come back when you're all better."

Does my family member first need to "hit rock bottom" before getting better?

No. Having an opioid addiction is painful, not only physically, but also emotionally. People with opioid addiction often are afraid of asking for help from those they love out of embarrassment, shame, disappointment in and anger toward themselves, and fear of abandonment. Even when family members see problems before the person with the addiction does, open and honest communication—in a caring, concerned, nonjudgmental, and non-threatening way—often helps the person to agree to seek help before the addiction progresses further.

Healthcare providers can also play a vital role in identifying and responding to early signs of addiction. Doctors, nurses, and physician assistants in primary care can screen for and diagnose opioid use disorder in their patients and start effective medications such as buprenorphine or injectable naltrexone.

Given the risk of fatal overdose with untreated addiction, waiting to help until someone "hits rock bottom" is not only unnecessary, but it also is very dangerous.

How can I cope with the stress of having a family member with opioid addiction?

There is a reason that addiction has been called a family disease: The strain affects everyone. The burden is financial, as families bear the cost of treatment or defense attorneys. It is interpersonal, as family members disagree on the best way to help. It is also deeply personal, as mothers, fathers, sisters, brothers, and children feel betrayed.

Ignoring these pressures is a mistake. Even as families are mobilizing to help a loved one with addiction, they should take steps to help themselves. These steps include talking over difficult decisions together with trusted clinicians, seeking sources of spiritual or psychological support (including counseling as needed), and joining non-judgmental family support groups. These groups help families understand that they are not struggling in isolation. Local clinicians and health departments can provide referrals in your area.

What is the role of home drug testing?

When someone with opioid addiction is living at home, family members, particularly parents, often are interested in monitoring the use of drugs. While home testing can sometimes be helpful for everyone involved, it is a practice that is also fraught with potential problems that threaten family relationships. Much of the friction around drug testing at home comes from fear. People with addiction are afraid of potential consequences—such as being told to immediately leave the house—that compound feelings of abandonment, worthlessness, guilt, and shame. Parents and other family members fear for the safety of the individual and themselves, even as they may feel anger, disappointment and hurt.

There are a few steps to consider.

First, before starting, families should talk with the person with the opioid addiction about the reasons for wanting to do the tests. Discussing this in a non-judgmental, factual, and caring way may cause less friction and conflict than with an accusatory tone. Using drug tests to "catch" a loved one doing something "wrong" does not foster an open, honest, or trusting relationship and may undermine the whole testing process.

Second, families should make a plan with the individual in case of positive results. The plan should include only those actions that family members agree will be implemented, and describe the order or circumstances in which they will occur.

This way, everyone knows up-front what to expect and when. A clear plan allows family members to model and maintain consistency and predictability in the face of the chaos addiction creates.

The plan should also reward honesty and openness. Here's a case example: A family makes a plan with their 29-year old daughter with an opioid addiction who is living at home. The plan includes a set of expectations including that if the daughter comes home and tells the parents she has used opioids before a drug test is done, the positive drug test will not result in her being asked to leave. Instead, it will result in a visit the next day to her addiction medicine doctor to discuss her treatment.

Third, families should recognize the limitations of drug tests. Someone who is using heroin will typically continue to have an opiate positive test for up to 3 days or so; testing every day or multiple times a day will not necessarily yield any additional information—just cause more friction. If a loved one says they have not used in 2 days but the test is still positive, he or she could very well be telling the truth. Similarly, families should recognize that drug testing is not perfect. If a loved one ate a poppy seed roll shortly before providing a urine specimen, the drug test might be opiate positive, and it would not be due to heroin. When there is any confusion about what a drug test means, families should talk to a healthcare provider.

How can I help a family member who is in recovery from opioid addiction?

A family's role is never over—not when opioid misuse starts, and not when it ends. Not even when affected family members return to work, or when they start a family. But the opportunities to help change.

The first opportunity to support recovery is to be liberal with words of encouragement and support. Rather than say, in anger, "I have never forgiven you for that time when you crashed my car," a family member might say, "I'm so impressed that you are taking each day at a time"—and wait for a calmer moment to talk about the car.

A second opportunity is to help the loved one avoid situations that may trigger a relapse. If someone in early recovery says, "I'd rather not go downtown to pick up the mail package, because that's where I used to go to get high," a family member might respond, "No problem. I'll get the package."

A third opportunity is to help with connections to effective treatment and support groups, including peer recovery services. Such services assist many people in making the transition back to a productive life.

A fourth opportunity is not to panic when family members early in recovery experience cravings in response to triggers encountered throughout their day. In fact, even years after their last use of alcohol or drugs, people may still experience cravings in response to significant stress.

When such cravings occur, families understandably may get anxious that a relapse is imminent. With that anxiety come all the painful memories and fears associated with past episodes. As a result, family members may become hypervigilant toward the person with addiction, setting up a vicious circle of suspicion and distrust.

A better approach is to talk over the situation and see what can be done to help. Talking through these anxieties and fears, with or without a health professional, can strengthen family relationships and alleviate some of the anxiety everyone is feeling—including the person with the addiction. In these situations, consistent support from family members may help protect against a relapse.

10

RECOVERY FROM OPIOID ADDICTION

What is recovery from opioid addiction?

Recovery is the process of moving beyond a pathological engagement with opioids. It includes such steps as rebuilding constructive relationships, establishing a stable living situation, and finding meaning and purpose in life. Every person has a different journey to recovery and, indeed, a different experience of its meaning. (Formal definitions are available in Appendix 3.)

The brains of individuals in recovery are, in a sense, healing. With greater maturity comes increased personal responsibility, an ability to look beyond oneself to the health and well-being of others, and a healthier approach to managing stressful life circumstances and emotions.

There is some debate about whether recovery requires total abstinence, with the prevailing view that any misuse of opioids puts someone at high risk for relapse.

There is also some confusion about whether it is possible for someone to be treated with medications and still be in recovery. The answer is yes: It very much is possible. Many people in recovery take medication for depression, bipolar disease, and other psychiatric and medical conditions, as well as for opioid addiction. With their medications, they have stopped misusing opioids, display no behaviors associated with addiction, are gainfully employed, own their own homes, have repaired family relationships, are involved in their faith communities, mentor others, and take care of their health. These are the hallmarks of recovery.

Here's a case example: A 29-year-old woman comes into a treatment program with a friend after 10 years of using heroin. She has dropped out of school, has endured periods of homelessness, and has lost her two children to foster care. She tells the treatment program that her primary goal is to get her kids back. Once she is receiving a therapeutic dose of methadone, she feels much better. She begins to work with her counselor to learn about what triggers her cravings to use heroin and how to cope with them. She completes her high school education and graduates from community college with a degree in counseling services. In the process, she regains custody of and raises her children. Twenty years later, her children are doing well as adults, and she still visits her treatment program once a month and picks up her methadone to take home. She works full time as a counselor and volunteers on weekends through her church, helping stock a food pantry for families experiencing homelessness.

What are 12-step programs?

Alcoholics Anonymous (AA) began in 1935 when Dr. Robert Smith and Bill Wilson, both in recovery from alcohol addiction, began reaching out to others with this condition. In 1939, Smith and Wilson held the first mutual support group meeting of AA and published the "Big Book, "which lays out the spiritually-grounded, 12 steps recommended as "a program of recovery."[1] Core elements of AA include mentorship from people in recovery, regular meetings, and testimony from individuals about how alcohol has affected their lives. Millions of people have benefitted from AA over the last 80 years.

The success of AA has led to the development of many other peer-led, recovery programs. These include Narcotics

Anonymous, focused on addiction to substances, including opioids; Celebrate Recovery, which has a religious focus; Women for Sobriety, focused on the unique needs of women; and Self-Management and Recovery Training (SMART), which is secular in orientation. Addiction treatment programs may host their own groups. Professional societies may sponsor groups just for their members, such as the medical profession for physicians with addiction.

Peer-led programs help many people, but these programs do not help everyone. Some people become intensely uncomfortable discussing addiction with peers and even find that such experiences trigger cravings and substance use. Nonetheless, enthusiasm for 12-step programs has led to a common misunderstanding that they are indispensable for everyone with an opioid addiction. Some judges order people to attend mutual support groups as part of a drug court program or a probation order, regardless of whether they are helpful. Some specialty addiction treatment programs and specialists require mutual support attendance as a prerequisite to receiving treatment or medication services without assessing if the patient is benefiting from them.

Another concern is that some 12-step programs reinforce stigma, particularly the stigma on medication treatment. Peer-led groups may not only mistakenly call the use of methadone and buprenorphine "addiction by another means" but also tell people that taking any medication for a mental health condition, such as depression, is a "cop-out." Writing in *The New Republic*, Katrine Jo Andersen and Cecile Maria Kallestrup told this story of an individual in recovery from opioid addiction named David:

As David walked back from the podium, he felt confused and alone. Should he trust his doctor, who had told him that [buprenorphine] was an effective way of treating opioid addiction and akin to an antidepressant? Or his peers, who preached complete abstinence, even from medication—and honesty, no secrets, as the only pathway to recovery? In the support group people had shared their darkest secrets as part of the 12 Steps to recovery. Some had told the group that they had been molested as children. One had even confessed to David that he had committed a murder. "But I didn't even feel comfortable to say that I was on [buprenorphine]," David said.[2]

Because the chance of relapse increases when people stop taking medications for opioid addiction, people who are bullied into dropping out of treatment can wind up overdosing and dying.

The bottom line is that peer-led recovery programs can be very helpful—so long as they respect and equally support everyone's path to recovery.

How can peers assist with recovery?

Aside from 12-step programs, peers can play a vital role in the recovery process.

Formally, people with a history of opioid addiction are increasingly taking jobs as recovery specialists or peer advocates. The development of these new types of positions is supported by federal and state agencies that recognize the valuable life experience that people in recovery can bring to others. Peer recovery specialists now typically receive special training and even acquire certification to provide services in a number of different settings. These include specialty addiction treatment programs, emergency departments, inpatient hospital wards, primary care offices, and even schools. The services peer recovery specialists provide range from emotional support, case management, other linkages to community-based recovery supports, and non-clinical recovery guidance in a safe, ethical, and authentic manner.[3]

For example, someone who experiences an opioid overdose in the state of Rhode Island is likely to meet a peer recovery specialist in the emergency department. The peer provides emotional support and helps the person develop a plan that may save their life.

Beyond these formal roles, peers—regardless of whether they have a history of addiction—can play a vital role in recovery. Many people with opioid addiction benefit from the support of classmates from school, co-workers at a job, and long-time childhood friends. Their consistent, healthy presence can help individuals in recovery through the ups and downs of life without the use of drugs or alcohol.

What kinds of supports do people in recovery need?

Recovery support services are as varied as the needs of the individuals who benefit from them. These include:

- Mutual support programs, such as 12-step programs, particularly those that do not discriminate against people who are taking medications for addiction treatment;
- Individual peer support services, such as emotional support and case management;
- Recovery drop-in centers, which provide a safe space for individuals to come to obtain a range of formal and informal supports;
- Recovery high schools and colleges, which provide a broad range of courses that help people complete their education in a safe, supportive environment free of alcohol and drugs or learn skills to rejoin the workforce;
- Employment training, which helps people find and succeed in jobs; and
- Recovery housing, which provides a safe and stable living environment.

The availability of these recovery services is growing, as the result of a sustained effort by the federal Substance Abuse and Mental Health Services Administration in collaboration with a number of national experts and organizations. Underlying these initiatives is a recognition that addiction is a chronic illness, without a known cure. Therefore, it makes sense to invest in supporting long-term recovery.

What is recovery housing?

Recovery housing refers to domestic settings in which a small group of people with addiction live together in a supportive alcohol and drug-free environment. Recovery housing has also been known as transitional housing or sober housing or living. There are no formal treatment services provided in recovery houses, but people who reside in them often attend specialty outpatient addiction treatment services.

Peer-run, independently operated, free-standing recovery houses have a long history in the United States, having grown out of the principles of AA. The first such houses started in California in the late 1940s as a place where people engaged in the AA 12 steps could safely live while they "worked their program."[4] Often located in neighborhoods where housing was cheap, sober houses required residents to adhere to strict rules of behavior and contribute financially to rent and other household bills. Entry into a sober living environment typically occurred through word of mouth as the operators and residents of the house tried to remain anonymous to the community around them. With strong stigma attached to addiction, communities typically were not eager to learn about the opening of a sober living house in their neighborhoods.

Today, there is a tremendous need for recovery housing to help individuals with opioid addiction. Two factors, however, are holding back the supply.

First, there is a wide range of quality in recovery housing. Because no treatment services are provided, recovery houses have historically not been regulated or overseen by state or federal agencies. As a result, some unscrupulous operators have taken advantage of vulnerable people early in recovery. There have been allegations of operators extorting their residents financially or sexually. Some homes have partnered with equally unscrupulous treatment providers and taken kickbacks from insurance claims for medically unnecessary drug testing and high-cost treatment services. Some have charged exorbitant rents in return for substandard living conditions.[5]

Second, many recovery housing programs refuse to accept individuals taking methadone and buprenorphine for addiction treatment. Some have adopted this rule as a matter of ideology; others assert that this is what the people who live in the house want for themselves. Either way, the result is that many people are forced to choose between effective treatment and a safe place to live.

Fortunately, federal and state lawmakers are beginning to take steps toward increasing oversight and regulation of recovery housing. The National Alliance of Recovery Residences, a non-profit organization formed in 2011, publishes a national standard and certification program for recovery houses that some states have implemented as a way of improving quality and reigning in poor practices. In addition, the Alliance promotes all recovery residence operators, staff, and volunteers to sign onto a code of ethics as part of best practices for recovery homes.[6] Unfortunately, these standards and codes do not explicitly bar discrimination against individuals receiving medication for addiction treatment.

What are threats to recovery?

Even people in long-term, stable recovery face a risk of relapse. Triggering events can be sudden, unexpected, and significant life stressors, such as getting fired from a job or the sudden death of a loved one.

Here's a case example: A man injects heroin regularly between the ages of 17 and 28, at which time he seeks treatment with methadone at the urging of his girlfriend. He quickly stabilizes in treatment, stops using heroin, begins making progress toward long-term recovery. He marries his girlfriend and works his way up to floor manager for a paint company over a 30-year career. With the support of his family, his work, and his friends, he manages his opioid addiction well until just before he is to retire from his job. By this time, he has stopped taking methadone, having slowly tapered off under medical supervision. Then, his wife dies suddenly of a heart attack. He is devastated. Despite all the support around him, he cannot cope with the grief. One day, an old acquaintance, who has stopped by to see how he was doing, hands him an oxycodone pill. The man takes it and within days is back to injecting heroin.

Factors that protect against relapse include safe and affordable housing, stable finances, access to needed physical and mental healthcare, a lack of outstanding legal problems, and strong social supports. Some people in long-term recovery describe having strong social supports as the most important protective factor out of this whole list. When people in recovery start to isolate themselves, lose touch with family and friends, or get overwhelmed and begin to doubt themselves—"go up in their head"—the risk of relapse increases.

Others in long-term recovery point to their involvement in positive activities as the factor that provides the most support. For them, filling their days with activities that provide meaning and purpose generates a sense of fulfillment that they perhaps may have sought through drugs or alcohol or lost while using. Joining other people with like-minded goals in these efforts also often leads to strong, healthy, supportive relationships that they can count on outside of any formal school, work, or other community setting.

How can addiction treatment providers support recovery?

Addiction treatment providers can help their patients achieve long-term success by aligning their services with the recovery process. This means paying attention to the broad spectrum of a person's needs and supporting, as much as possible, recovery-related activities. For instance, learning how to celebrate happy occasions without drugs and alcohol can be a challenge for people with addiction. Treatment programs can assist by hosting events such as a substance-free holiday meal or a Super Bowl Sunday party. Some treatment providers have organized movie outings and dance recitals.

Clinic policies should support recovery, not hinder it. This means working with patients who have difficulty coming to clinic on particular days as a result of changing work schedules. It means scheduling parents with small children and inadequate childcare for individual counseling sessions and allowing them to bring their young ones to clinic. And it means thinking outside of the usual brick-and-mortar building to reach people with services—whether through telemedicine, adding peers to help with outreach in the community, and having formal connections with entities that provide vocational training, employment, housing, and mutual support.

To better coordinate treatment and recovery, some in the addiction field are now calling for the development not just of treatment plans, but of recovery plans. Such plans should include specific goals and actions the person has identified to help them achieve and sustain recovery. Healthcare providers can use these recovery plans as part of recovery check-ups over time, just as people with hypertension get their blood pressure checked at regular intervals.

Section 3

COMMUNITIES AND POLICY

11

A HISTORICAL PERSPECTIVE ON THE OPIOID EPIDEMIC

When did the opioid epidemic start?

Some point to January 10, 1980, as the first day of America's opioid epidemic. That's when the *New England Journal of Medicine* published a one-paragraph letter with the title "Addiction Rare in Patients Treated with Narcotics."[1] Over the next 25 years, the letter would be cited hundreds of times as part of a movement to expand the use of opioids for the treatment of chronic pain.

The letter's author, Boston University Professor Hershel Jick, would later state that he was "mortified" about his letter's legacy, as his research related to hospitalized patients, not patients with chronic pain.[2] Nevertheless, the rate of opioid prescribing jumped more than fourfold over the next three decades,[3] with increasing numbers of patients requesting larger doses, craving the medications, and using them despite all sorts of harms—the hallmarks of addiction.

Others trace the start of the epidemic to an earlier point in US history. A much earlier point. During the Civil War, physicians began using opioids to treat thousands suffering from the injuries of battle. Opioid use also became increasingly common among upper-class women for a variety of ailments, real and imagined.

William Faulkner wrote, "The past is never dead. It's not even past."[4] This statement applies particularly well to the US history with opioids. From the 1890s to the 1980s, our nation passed through four distinct stages:

1. Overprescribing for pain (late 19th century);
2. A clampdown on opioid use in medicine (early 20th century);
3. The rising use of illicit opioids (mid-20th century); and
4. A conflicted response, including both greater access to treatment and strong criminal penalties (late 20th century).

With eerie similarities, what happened over a century ago has also repeated itself over the last several decades: the overprescribing of opioids for pain, followed by a clampdown, the rising use of illicit opioids, and, most recently, a response that mixes treatment with law enforcement. Meanwhile, the toll of the epidemic has risen to unprecedented levels.

George Santayana said, "Those who cannot remember the past are condemned to repeat it."[5] Ever since the late 19th century, there have been individuals who have sought to address opioid use in the United States as a public health problem— people who have recognized the benefits and risks of opioids for pain, the chronic nature of addiction and the value of treatment that helps people regain control over their lives. However, public health approaches have always struggled to become the dominant responses to the opioid epidemic.

Will this time be different?

Why have historians called the opioid problem "The American Disease"?

Even before the United States was formed as a nation, physicians and others in the healing professions relied on opioids to provide pain relief; 17th-century English physician Thomas Sydenham called opium "one of the most valued medicines in the world [that] does more honor to medicine than any remedy whatsoever."[6] The history of opioids in the United States is accordingly as old as the republic; opium is said to have soothed Alexander Hamilton as he lay dying after his duel with Aaron Burr.[7]

America's unique problem with opioids can be traced to the Civil War. Since that time, no other country has experienced the same challenges with opioid addiction. In the early years, these struggles evolved in four stages—stages that will resonate as familiar to those observing today's opioid epidemic.

Stage 1: Overprescribing for pain

In response to the injuries of Civil War battles, US physicians increased their use of opioids to treat pain. Nearly 10 million opium pills and 2.8 million ounces of tinctures and powders were provided to Union soldiers alone.[8] Soldiers who survived the war often found their way to those physicians armed with a new tool of the trade—the hypodermic needle. Long-term use of opioids began to be known as "soldier's disease" or "army disease."

In the latter half of the 19th century, physicians began to prescribe opioids more frequently to middle-class and upper-class women. A leading gynecology textbook in 1865 stated that opium was an "energetic palliative treatment" for menstrual cramps, and other guides recommended opioids for a long list of "female complaints." One observer would write that "uterine and ovarian complications cause more ladies to fall into the habit, than all other diseases combined."[9]

As prescriptions increased, some patients started demanding increasing doses and neglected their other responsibilities. By 1898, the gynecology textbook had changed its tune to read, "He who is compelled to resort frequently to opium and stimulants" for menstrual cramps "must be considered devoid in diagnostic ability, and consequently ought not to be entrusted with the management of such cases."[10] A public policy response was not far behind.

Stage 2: A clampdown on opioid use in medicine

By the end of the 19th century, several US states had begun to take steps to limit opioid use. The first set of actions limited the over-the-counter sale of opioids. These laws, however, provided an exception for opioids included in custom remedies known as patent medicines. Mrs. Winslow's Soothing Syrup for Infants, for example, contained as much as 65 mg of morphine per fluid ounce.[11]

By the early 20th century, with estimates of "habitual users" of opioids as high as 250,000, concern about overprescribing of opioids led to a tightening of restrictions on manufacturers and prescribers. In 1903, a group established by the American Pharmaceutical Association, called the Committee on the Acquirement of the Drug Habit, released a report calling for strong federal action. The report stated, "The murderer who destroys a man's body is an angel beside one who destroys that man's soul and mind."[12]

In 1906, Congress passed and President Theodore Roosevelt signed the Pure Food and Drugs Act, which required manufacturers of remedies and medications to list several key ingredients, including opioids, on the label. This did not solve the problem. In 1908, the president appointed "a handsome doctor with a handlebar mustache" as the nation's first opioid commissioner. Dr. Hamilton Wright told the *New York Times*: "The habit has this nation in its grip to an astonishing extent. . . . Our prisons and our hospitals are full of victims of it, it has robbed ten thousand businessmen of moral sense and made them beasts who prey upon their fellows . . . it has become one of the most fertile causes of unhappiness and sin in the United States."[13] Anti-opioid efforts culminated in the 1914 passage of the Harrison Act, which established a broad regulatory structure that included registration and taxation of opioids. It also required that opioids be available to patients only by prescription, and only with prescriptions written "in good faith"—a term that was not defined.

Authorities enforced the new law fiercely. Thousands of physicians were arrested and prosecuted for, in the words of one court, the "gratification of a diseased appetite for these pernicious drugs."[14,15] Ruthless enforcement in the medical system carried over into law enforcement efforts against heroin and other illicit opioids. Over the ensuing several decades, police arrested tens of thousands of people who used opioids, and judges sent them to large penal "narcotic farms" in the Midwest. In 1956, Congress passed the Narcotic Control Act, which included the first mandatory minimum sentences for a first conviction of possession—as well as the death penalty for drug trafficking.

Stage 3: A rise in illicit opioids

Despite the crackdown, underground opioid use never disappeared. In 1960 in New York City, heroin overdose was the leading cause of death among young adults between the ages of 15 and 35.[16] Then, with cultural changes sweeping the nation and the protests against the Vietnam War, the use of illicit drugs—including heroin—increased again substantially. Historian David Musto has estimated that the number of heroin users increased tenfold from 1960 to 1970, from 50,000 to 500,000.[17]

Stage 4: A mixed response

On June 17, 1971, President Richard M. Nixon issued a special message to Congress about the "tide of drug abuse that has swept America in the last decade." In this message, considered the launch of the war on drugs, the president set out a series of actions to address both the supply of and demand for illicit drugs.[18]

To reduce the availability of heroin, Nixon increased efforts to block its import, imposed greater penalties on drug sellers, and sped up the "prosecution of narcotic trafficking cases."

The announcement went beyond enforcement measures. To reduce interest in using heroin, the president set a national goal "to destroy the market for drugs, and this means the prevention of new addicts, and the rehabilitation of those who are addicted." Nixon established a network of clinics that offered treatment with a newly appreciated medication, methadone. In fact, the first budget for the war on drugs set aside about two-thirds of the funding for treatment. The major investment in treatment had an immediate impact. Areas of the country where people received care reported lower overdose rates and less crime. FBI crime statistics for 1972 found a 3% reduction in crime nationally, the first decline in nearly two decades.

Yet despite the initial success of "demand reduction," the enforcement side of the war on drugs came to dominate the nation's response. By the time President Reagan took office in 1981, there had been a vast increase in resources for drug interdiction abroad and law enforcement at home. Then the 1986 Anti-Drug Abuse Act provided additional billions for policing and imposed mandatory minimum sentencing at the federal level for minor drug offenses. Many states added their own mandatory minimum sentences. These laws led directly to the explosive growth of the nation's jails and prisons, filled disproportionately with urban residents and racial and ethnic minorities.

It was in this context that a movement started to provide better care for patients in pain—including by encouraging the greater use of opioids for a growing list of short-term and chronic conditions.

The cycle had begun again.

What led to the increase in prescriptions of opioids for pain from 1990 to 2010?

For many decades after the passage of the Harrison Act in 1914, physicians rarely prescribed opioid medications for chronic use. Doing so would have invited prosecution. The law limited the use of opioids to prescriptions in good faith, and courts did not recognize long-term prescriptions to "habitual users" as a legitimate medical practice.[19]

And then, starting in the 1980s, the culture of medicine began to change.

Part of the road to change was paved with good intentions—particularly the goal of better treating pain. National surveys showed a rising incidence of pain, attributed to the aging of the population and a greater number of people surviving with chronic illnesses and injuries. Studies showed that African Americans were less likely to receive pain medications for long-bone fractures and African Americans, Hispanic Americans, and Asian Americans were less likely to receive treatment for chronic pain associated with cancer.[20] Patient advocacy groups and a vocal group of clinicians began demanding the medical profession "move beyond the stigma attached to opioid use and worries about addiction and recognize the drugs' value for patients with intractable pain."[21]

The push to prescribe more opioids for pain had powerful allies in the pharmaceutical companies that began marketing a new generation of long acting opioids. The largest was Purdue Pharma, the manufacturer of OxyContin®, introduced to the market in 1996. One potential advantage of this pill was convenience; it combined the opioid oxycodone with a slow-release technology so it could be dosed twice a day compared to four times a day for the generic version. But this modest difference was enough to support an enormous marketing campaign.

Purdue spent hundreds of millions of dollars selling OxyContin® to physicians. According to one report, "from 1996 to 2001, Purdue conducted more than 50 national pain-management and speaker-training conferences at resorts in Florida, Arizona, and California. More than 5000 physicians, pharmacists and nurses attended these all-expenses-paid symposia, where they were recruited and trained for Purdue's national speaker bureau."[22] Purdue tracked the prescribing of individual physicians and gave out tens of millions of bonuses to sales representatives who could drive up the number of prescriptions. To physicians and nurses, Purdue distributed thousands of "fishing hats, stuffed plush toys and music compact discs" branded "Get in the Swing with OxyContin"; to their patients, Purdue provided coupons that covered their first OxyContin® prescriptions. The campaign was spectacularly successful. Sales of OxyContin® grew to more than $1 billion annually within 5 years, with more than 6.2 million prescriptions written in 2002.[23]

A critical part of Purdue's success was minimizing concerns about addiction. Purdue extensively cited data out of context— quoting, for example, safety information derived from short-term use to reassure physicians about the safety of long-term use. The company also convinced the US Food and Drug Administration to include in the drug's label that the long-acting nature of OxyContin® made the medication much less likely to cause addiction. This point turned out not to be true; many who originally received the medication for pain became addicted.

The cultural change in prescribing opioids for pain touched every corner of medical practice—from cardiology to neurology, from dentistry to emergency medicine, from nurse practitioners to physician assistants, and from surgery to primary care.[24] General practitioners came to account for about half of all prescription opioids provided to patients.[25]

Enthusiasm for prescribing opioids for pain penetrated every corner of the nation's medical system, from big cities to rural communities. Emergency room doctors invented the term "oligoanalgesia" to describe inadequate pain treatment as a medical symptom.[26] In 1996, the American Pain Society adopted the concept of pain as reported by the patient as a fifth vital sign, a paradigm then adopted by the Veterans Health Administration in 1998.[27] In 2000, the Joint Commission on Accreditation of Healthcare Organizations began to use pain control as a key element of inspections of hospitals.

Federal health agencies facilitated this shift. The Food and Drug Administration permitted Purdue and other companies to market their products for "long-term use" despite the lack of studies examining opioids' long-term effects, and the Centers for Medicare and Medicaid Services began to assess how healthcare facilities and their clinicians responded to patients' complaints of pain. Many doctors feared the consequences of a drop in patient satisfaction scores if they refused requests for opioid pain medications.

As late as 2011, the Institute of Medicine, the nation's most prestigious medical authority, released a report declaring pain a public health crisis in the country, affecting more than 100 million Americans. The report suggested opioids were still underutilized and blamed reports of addiction on the "misdeeds or carelessness" of certain physicians and patients.[28] At the time this report was published, the most commonly prescribed medication in the United States was the opioid hydrocodone, at about 130 million prescriptions each year,[29] and the United States was consuming about 80% of the world's supply of prescription opioids.[30]

As the prescribing of opioids doubled in the United States, and then doubled again, three unfortunate patterns began to come into focus. First, many clinicians prescribed too many opioids for short-term pain. After minor procedures such as wisdom tooth extraction, many patients went home with a month or more of opioids, when a couple days (at most) would have sufficed. These extra medications could be borrowed or stolen by others and contribute to addiction and risk of overdose. Second, some doctors opened "pill mills" where they fraudulently wrote prescriptions, often in return for cash payments, for large amounts of opioids without a legitimate evaluation of the patient and with no meaningful follow-up. Third, many clinicians, particularly primary care doctors, began to prescribe greater amounts of opioids for chronic non-cancer pain and for longer periods of time. This third path would prove to be the greatest source of the increase in opioid prescribing—and to be particularly difficult to address.

What was the response to the overprescription of opioids?

In 1919, facing the problem of opioid overprescribing by the medical community, the New York City Health Commissioner offered a simple policy recommendation: the physicians who were responsible "should be boiled in oil."[31] Nearly a century later, a similar frustration and anger—in spirit, if not in words—returned.

The pushback began in the early 2000s, when some physicians started to question the increased use of opioid medications. In a 2003 article in the *New England Journal of Medicine* (one that has aged particularly well), Dr. Jane C. Ballantyne and Dr. Jiaren Mao wrote that "high-dose opioid therapy may be neither safe nor effective." Citing evidence that the benefits of the medications can wear off over time, leaving patients with increasing risks of adverse effects including addiction, they recommended that "physicians make every effort to control indiscriminate prescribing, even when they are under pressure by patients to increase the dose of opioids."[32]

Other physicians began to object to aggressive marketing by pharmaceutical companies. One pain management physician in Bangor, Maine, told the *New York Times* that he threw a Purdue Pharma representative out of his office for "pushing [OxyContin®] for everything."[33] At a 2003 debate at a medical meeting, later reported in the *Journal of the American Medical Association*, one physician stated, "What we don't know is the real downside of these medications, which have been blithely dismissed by the academic zealots and brushed aside by the manufacturers."[34]

Reports soon surfaced about patients lining up at pain management clinics for prescriptions,[35] overdose fatalities increasing,[36] and illicit markets forming for the diversion and misuse of OxyContin®.[37] By the end of 2001, both *48 Hours* and MTV's *True Life* series had broadcast the stories of people crushing and snorting or injecting OxyContin® to defeat its slow-release technology.[38] Misuse of opioids began to rise dramatically in rural areas, where pharmaceutical distributors were sending millions of tablets of pain medication.

Next came a range of legal actions. As early as 2002, state prosecutors in Florida and elsewhere began to pursue criminal charges against physicians whose patients died of overdoses.[39] The West Virginia attorney general charged Purdue Pharma for downplaying the risks of OxyContin® addiction; the company settled the case for $10 million in 2004.[40] Three years later, Purdue pled guilty to criminal charges brought by the US Department of Justice and paid more than $600 million in fines. Then, under pressure by the US Food and Drug Administration, Purdue reformulated OxyContin® to make the pills more difficult to crush.[41] As overdose deaths continued to mount, more states and localities began to file suit against Purdue and other opioid manufacturers, seeking billions in damages.

There were also efforts to target fraudulent and unethical prescribing. In 2010, Florida began shutting down clinics dubbed "pill mills" for distributing millions of doses of opioids to out-of-state residents indiscriminately; the Florida attorney general stated the goal was to prosecute "the drug dealers wearing white coats."[42]

To identify patients who sought and received prescriptions from opioid medications from multiple doctors, states began to set up—with federal government funding—large databases called Prescription Drug Monitoring Programs. These databases included records of every controlled substance prescription, so that doctors could find patients searching for and receiving opioids from multiple prescribers.

Eventually, it became clear that the problem was not just with the rogue company, or the unethical physician, or even the troubled patient. The finger of blame began to point at the culture of medicine itself. By 2010, levels of opioid prescribing had risen to three or four times that of any other country in the world. The problem touched thousands upon thousands of clinicians who had come to believe their job was to better treat pain by using opioids.

Efforts to change medical practice followed. In 2013, then Massachusetts Governor Deval Patrick tried to ban the sale of a new, long-acting opioid medication in his state. Massachusetts and other states began to pass laws limiting initial opioid prescriptions to several days. National associations including the American Academy of Family Physicians revised guidelines for the use of opioids for the treatment of pain,[43] and in 2016, the Centers for Disease Control and Prevention (CDC) published the first-ever national standard for the use of opioids in the management of chronic, non-cancer pain by primary care practitioners.[44] Among other steps, the CDC guideline recommended non-pharmacological treatment such as physical therapy first, with carefully monitored opioid use as a last resort. The CDC review, and a 2014 review from the Agency for Healthcare Research and Quality, had failed to find any studies demonstrating the effectiveness of opioid use past a few weeks.

These efforts have had an impact on prescribing. From a peak in 2010, prescriptions for opioids fell 33% by 2017—but still remained more than 4 times higher than the amount prescribed in 1992.[45] The attention to clinical practice also triggered a wave of introspection. "We as a profession have caused an epidemic that is bigger than the HIV epidemic," noted physician and author Atul Gawande said at a public forum in 2017, "We started it."[46]

By 2017, however, it was too late for the medical profession to fix the problem by more judicious prescribing of opioids for pain alone. The recent epidemic might have started with irrational exuberance for prescription opioid use, but by this point, a critical shift had taken place. As had happened a century earlier, efforts to rein in prescribing were followed by a different kind of opioid challenge.

*Have tighter regulations on opioid prescriptions
contributed to a rise in use of heroin?*

Yes, but it's complicated.

In 2007, 399 Maryland residents died of a heroin-related overdose, a relatively large number that reflected the popularity of the drug in the state. This toll then fell over the next few years, so that by 2011, heroin claimed the lives of just 247 Marylanders. Then, in 2012, there were 392 deaths from heroin—leading the state to issue a public health advisory.

It would keep getting worse. In 2013, Maryland experienced 464 heroin overdose deaths—the most on record— and it became clear the Old Line State was far from alone. In July of that year, *The New York Times* reported that "heroin, which has long flourished in the nation's big urban centers, has been making an alarming comeback in the smaller cities and towns of New England."[47] The CDC would later report that from 2000 to 2013, the death rate from heroin nearly quadrupled—with the largest increase seen in the Midwest.[48]

That heroin deaths were spiking as the number of prescriptions for opioids were starting to decline was not entirely a coincidence. Some patients shifted from pharmaceutical medications like OxyContin® to illicit forms of opioids like heroin. Indeed, the CDC would later report that people addicted to prescription opioids were 40 times more likely to become addicted to heroin than the rest of the population.[49]

Stories of the transition from opioid medications to heroin began to surface. Dr. Sanjay Gupta reported on *CNN*, "It is precisely because there are so many similarities that pain pill addicts frequently turn to heroin when pills are no longer available to them."[50] One 17-year old told *The New York Times* that when OxyContin® became too expensive, the obvious choice to was to turn to heroin. She said, "My parents had no idea. . . . Who would've thought that such a bad drug could be so easily accessible to me?"[51] Author Sam Quinones, in his compelling book *Dreamland*, described a ready market for Mexican heroin in small cities and towns across America where opioid prescribing had increased dramatically.[52]

However, there was more to the rise in heroin than the decline in prescription opioid prescribing. For one, the increase in heroin use started in some areas before prescribing began to plateau and decline. For another, those states that took greater action on prescribing did not see the greatest increases in heroin deaths; in these areas, reducing inappropriate prescribing may have kept some people from developing an opioid addiction in the first place.[53]

The United States quickly found itself facing two problems at once, with multiple connections between them. Millions more Americans were receiving long-term opioid treatment for pain than ever before, with substantial numbers developing an addiction. At precisely the wrong point in time, unprecedented quantities of cheap heroin were entering the country from Afghanistan, Mexico, and other countries.

It was a perfect storm. The new heroin epidemic undermined any sense of relief from a slowing rate of opioid prescribing. On Staten Island, New York, for example, health officials reported a 29% decline in prescription opioid deaths from 2011 to 2013.[54] But the number of total deaths did not decline. Because of an increase in deaths from heroin, Staten Island soon had the highest rate of drug overdose death of any borough in New York City.[55]

Just when it seemed the problem could not possibly get any worse, something happened to make it much, much worse. Back in Maryland, after 464 people died from heroin in 2013, 578 died in 2014. Then, a shocking 748 Marylanders died from heroin overdoses in 2015. And a staggering 1,212 died in 2016.

The reason for this spike? Heroin was not just heroin anymore.

What is the fentanyl crisis?

Fentanyl is a highly potent opioid—1 unit has the same effect as about 50 units of morphine. In the hospital, carefully controlled amounts of fentanyl are used for anesthesia. Many young doctors learn to write prescriptions for tiny amounts of drugs using fentanyl as an example—writing mCg for a microgram, which is a thousand times smaller than a milligram. On the street, just a few grains of fentanyl gives the same effect as a thumb-sized vial of heroin.

The recent opioid epidemic in the United States has had three waves: the first, prescription opioids; the second, heroin; and the third, fentanyl.

With respect to overdose deaths, the third wave is the biggest of them all.

The first US brush with fentanyl came in the mid-2000s. On April 21, 2006, users of illicit drugs in Camden, New Jersey, started dying. Overdoses also spiked in Baltimore, Chicago, Detroit, and Philadelphia. A subsequent investigation by the CDC and the Drug Enforcement Administration turned up a specific culprit: non-pharmaceutical fentanyl had found its way into the supply of heroin and cocaine. Over 2 years, more than 1,000 Americans died.[56]

Then, law enforcement officials identified and shut down a lab making fentanyl in Toluca, Mexico. And the deaths stopped. Illicit fentanyl essentially disappeared from the United States for the next six years.

In November 2013, like a light switch coming back on, non-pharmaceutical fentanyl returned. Rhode Island issued the first warning,[57] with Maryland not far behind.[58] Public health officials hoped that fentanyl's return would be again be a temporary blip on the screen. But the problem only worsened. Fentanyl began to appear in an ever-expanding geographic radius, in increasing amounts and more than a dozen synthesized varieties. These included acetyl fentanyl, furofentanyl, and carfentanil, otherwise known as elephant tranquilizer.

The 2017 national threat assessment of the Drug Enforcement Administration found that fentanyl "is now widely available throughout the United States"[59]—sold with heroin or cocaine, pressed into counterfeit pills or sold alone. The motive is thought to be economic; the *Wall Street Journal* reported that just 25 grams of fentanyl costs $800 to produce and has an estimated street value of $800,000.[60] This makes fentanyl a much greater value for dealers than those illicit drugs (such as heroin, marijuana, and cocaine) that depend on agriculture. Labs in China and Mexico are suspected of producing fentanyl and its analogues, which then are mixed into other types of illicit drugs at various stages of the production and distribution process. Because fentanyl is so potent, an uneven mixing process can leave some of the drug supply without any meaningful amount of fentanyl and the rest more concentrated—and lethal.

Despite intense efforts, law enforcement have not as yet been able to stop the supply of fentanyl. The Drug Enforcement Agency has reported that "the original supplier in China will provide the package to a freight forwarding company or individual, who transfers it to another freight forwarder, who then takes custody and presents the package to customs for export."[61] This "makes it difficult for law enforcement to track these packages." With thousands of packages entering the country each day, law enforcement officials are concerned about the ability to disrupt the supply.

And that's not the only concern. Unlike with heroin—which drug users were seeking to buy—fentanyl is often hidden in the drug supply. Drug users may have no idea they are about to take a substance where the lethal dose is measured in micrograms. Taking a regular dose of drugs—but now adulterated with fentanyl—is a game of Russian roulette. Many emergency medical technicians have reported finding people dead before even consuming their entire dose. The performing artist Prince allegedly died from a fentanyl overdose associated with counterfeit prescription drugs,[62] as did Tom Petty.[63]

In large areas of the Northeast and Midwest, in just a few short years, fentanyl went from nowhere on the radar screen to a leading cause of death to *the* leading cause of death to the cause of *the majority* of deaths. By 2017, nearly 30,000 Americans died of overdoses associated with illicit fentanyl, up from virtually none 4 years earlier. Fentanyl was also responsible for a telling milestone, pushing the number of deaths from illicit opioids above the number from prescription opioids.

What started with an increase in prescribing for pain has led, as it did a century earlier, to a more dangerous—and far more complicated-- challenge. And yet again, our nation's response has been a conflicted mix of greater access to treatment and more intense enforcement.

What role has race played in the opioid epidemic?

In 1903, W. E. B. Dubois predicted that "the problem of the 20th century would be the problem of the color line."[64] Over the next 100 years, the United States' struggle with race intersected time and again with the "American disease" of opioid addiction. That's because, in the apt explanation of historian David Courtwright, "what we think about addiction very much depends on who is addicted."[65]

At the time Dr. Dubois was writing his famous words on race, white women were common consumers of opioid drugs, with their doctors the main suppliers. Many looked like Mrs. Henry Lafayette Dubose, the strange widow in Harper Lee's novel *To Kill a Mockingbird*, who took morphine for years after falling ill with a chronic condition. Others consumed opioids to relieve the drudgery of a world in which women were not permitted to pursue their education. As one woman of the early 20th century wrote, "you don't know what morphine means to some of us, many of us, modern women without professions, without beliefs. Morphine makes life possible."[66]

As the prescribing of opioids declined in response to concerns about addiction, the picture of the opioid user changed. Out went the image of the innocent white woman with a pill or a needle; in came the sinister visage of a Chinese man with a pipe. A professional task force established by the American Pharmaceutical Association at the turn of the 20th century announced, "If the Chinaman cannot get along without his 'dope,' we can get along without him."[67] The first U.S. law restricting the use of opioids, passed in 1909, prohibited only the importation and possession of opium processed for smoking, which was, not coincidentally, the preferred method of consumption of Chinese immigrants. It was called the Smoking Opium Exclusion Act.

Over the next decade, opioid use moved further to the margins of society. As prescriptions continued to fall, opioids became even more linked to people who were homeless, unemployed, or engaged in crime—in the words of one historian, to "foreigners and alien subgroups."[68]

The policy response was unforgiving. The 1914 Harrison Act not only turned many users into criminals but it also forbade physicians from prescribing the most effective forms of treatment—stable doses of opioids. As far back as the 1910s, it was well recognized that prescribing a maintenance dose of morphine or other opioids to long-time users in a stable manner allowed them to continue to function in society. A public health clinic in Jacksonville, Florida, for example, provided regular doses of opioids to registered individuals as part of a comprehensive plan for the early 20th-century opioid epidemic.[69] (The program even monitored area physicians for overprescribing.) Around the same time, in New York, a group of physicians argued "one of the first duties of the state, in dealing with this grave situation, [is] to establish a supply of narcotic drugs, to which the confirmed addict shall have access, under proper state regulation."[70]

Strident enforcers of the Harrison Act, however, went to court to close these programs. New federal law enforcement agencies, including the Bureau of Narcotics, arrested treating physicians and sent thousands of people who continued using drugs to large "narcotic farms" and pursued ever harsher punishments, including the death penalty. The view of addiction as a medical condition virtually disappeared.

This draconian approach finally started to wane in the 1960s, as, not coincidentally, the counterculture drew in more middle- and upper-class youth. Around this time, physicians and public health officials gained traction in their objections to penalties on people who used drugs and their advocacy for treatment, including the use of the medication methadone. The declaration in 1971 by President Nixon of a war on drugs included support for both treatment and law enforcement approaches, with investments in new services and research alongside aggressive action against the drug trade, particularly in US cities.

Then, in the 1980s, increases in cocaine use among African Americans led to a sharp resurgence in the stigma on drug use—and a dramatic acceleration in the use of force to suppress it. Congress passed and President Ronald Reagan signed laws with mandatory minimum sentences for drug possession, later shown to have a profound and disparate impact on African Americans and their communities. In response to the resulting urban devastation, Baltimore Mayor Kurt Schmoke asked in the early 1990s whether viewing addiction as a public health problem and offering drug treatment instead of incarceration might be a more effective approach. National politicians and the media pilloried Schmoke for being soft on crime.

Discussion of today's opioid epidemic remains tinged by race. As predominantly white areas of rural and suburban

America were affected by addiction to pain medication, a wave of compassion swept through the rhetoric of many politicians. 2016 Republican Presidential candidates Carly Fiorina, Chris Christie, and Jeb Bush all spoke movingly of friends and family who struggled with addiction. With broad bipartisan support, since 2016, Congress has appropriated several billion dollars to increase access to addiction treatment.

Yet, simultaneously, the recent spike in heroin and fentanyl deaths has led to a resurgence of aggressive strategies to address the drug supply. President Trump has blamed Mexico and Mexicans for drug imports and promised that a wall at the border and more aggressive use of the death penalty for drug trafficking would help reduce the problem. Several members of Congress have attempted to pin the opioid crisis on immigration and "sanctuary cities."[71] A new wave of mandatory minimum sentencing legislation related to fentanyl is passing state legislatures. As if to remind everyone that repugnant stereotypes are never too far out of reach, Maine Governor Paul LePage erroneously blamed 90% of drug trafficking in his state on individuals who are African American or Hispanic. He stated,

> "The traffickers—these aren't people who take drugs. These are guys by the name D-Money, Smoothie, Shifty. . . . These type of guys that come from Connecticut and New York. They come up here, they sell their heroin, then they go back home. . . . Incidentally, half the time they impregnate a young, white girl before they leave."[72]

Opioid use remains highly stigmatized in the United States. Patients receiving opioid medications for pain often fear that physicians will stop prescribing their treatment, and users of street opioids in cities and rural areas alike, regardless of race, often struggle to find effective treatment, to stay out of jail, and to find a path back to a normal life. This path remains particularly difficult for those experiencing racism and other forms of discrimination. As US policy has moved through a painfully familiar series of stages, the death toll has risen to new levels.

Making major progress with a public health approach will require both smart policy to address the overprescribing of opioids for pain as well as to expand access to needed services. Success will require not only following evidence but also learning the lessons of history.

12

PREVENTION POLICY FOR
THE OPIOID EPIDEMIC

How can communities prevent opioid addiction?

Addiction involves an interaction between the substance, an individual, and the environment. This means there are three ways to prevent addiction: by reducing exposure, by helping individuals remain resilient even when exposure occurs, and by promoting a healthy environment for all.

Progress on each of these fronts requires effective national and state policy as well as efforts within communities to effect change. In this sense, "community" refers to the residents, health professionals, and public officials of neighborhoods, cities, towns, and counties. All can make a difference.

Does reducing the excessive prescribing
of opioids prevent opioid addiction?

Yes. Only those patients who really need opioids should receive them—and in appropriate doses, too. Communities can embrace several approaches to promote appropriate prescribing and reduce the chance of misuse and addiction.

Make alternatives to opioids more available

Many patients with pain do not need opioids at all. Physical therapy, acupuncture, massage therapy, and counseling can all help many patients address chronic pain without the need for medications.[1] Unfortunately, as reported by the *New York Times*, "opioid drugs are generally cheap while safer alternatives are more expensive."[2] Insurers typically cover prescriptions for a low-cost opioid without any hurdles, but place extra steps or even hard limits on access to other types of therapies. Given the risks of unnecessary opioid use, these coverage decisions are unfortunate and shortsighted. Local employers and public officials at all levels of government can encourage (or even require) public and private insurers to offer broad coverage of non-pharmaceutical and non-opioid treatments for pain.

Better train prescribers

Many physicians and nurse practitioners have received little or no formal education in basic aspects of opioid prescribing, from deciding whether to prescribe to how best to monitor clinical improvement. Some state medical boards have added requirements for all practicing physicians; Georgia, for example, now requires 3 hours of training as a condition of license renewal.[3] In April 2018, Food and Drug Administration (FDA) Commissioner Dr. Scott Gottlieb suggested that the Drug Enforcement Administration could require special training as a condition of receiving a license to prescribe controlled substances.[4]

Unfortunately, professional medical associations often oppose these requirements; in Maryland, the state medical society in 2015 lobbied the general assembly and governor to overturn a requirement for just 1 hour of training every 2 years established by the Board of Medicine.[5] (The requirement was reinstated for prescribers of controlled substances 2 years later.)

Limit new prescriptions

There is growing evidence that for initial prescriptions, doctors prescribe more opioids—and in many cases, far more opioids—than patients need. Researchers study this question by assessing the frequency of refills. If virtually all patients who receive prescriptions for 2 days do not refill their medications, the researchers conclude that 2 days is just fine. Using this approach, the FDA found that for routine surgical procedures, many doctors prescribe 20 to 30 times more pills than patients need.[6] In 2016, Massachusetts became the first state to limit the length of new opioid prescriptions to 7 days.[7] Other states soon followed, although these laws have yet to be evaluated.

Promote evidence-based guidelines

Despite the recent emergence of expert recommendations on judicious practice, opioid prescribing in the United States remains threefold higher than opioid prescribing in other countries. Professional organizations and insurers can track whether clinicians follow these guidelines, including the Centers for Disease Control (CDC) guidelines for chronic, non-cancer pain, and follow up with those who do not. OptumLabs convened experts and developed 29 ways that insurers can measure appropriate treatment using insurance claims records.[8]

What are prescription drug monitoring programs?

Prescription drug monitoring programs are databases that include information on prescriptions of controlled substances. These databases can help prevent harm from prescription opioids in three ways.

First, prescribers can check at the time of a clinical visit to see whether their patients are receiving opioids from multiple sources—a warning sign for misuse. If a problem is found, prescribers should evaluate and refer their patients if appropriate, to treatment. Failing to do so may lead some people who are refused prescription opioids to turn to illicit markets for opioids, increasing their risk. Second, health officials can spot clinicians who show signs of prescribing opioids inappropriately. It is possible to offer these prescribers education, known as "academic detailing," to help them provide better clinical care. In more severe cases, states can place prescribers on probation or even remove their ability to prescribe controlled substances altogether. In extreme cases, where fraud appears likely, states can refer prescribers to medical boards (which might take their licenses away) or even to the Drug Enforcement Administration (which can prosecute them under federal law).

Third, policymakers can assess whether prescribing on the whole is improving. Are clinicians in a county or state starting opioids in new patients for just a few days, or are longer prescriptions more common? Are patients being prescribed opioids along with benzodiazepines, a combination that increases the risk for breathing problems and overdose? How frequently are patients receiving a dose of opioids that is associated with a higher risk of overdose? Are patients receiving opioids for chronic pain also receiving prescriptions for naloxone to have on hand in case of overdose? The data in prescription drug monitoring programs can answer these and other questions to inform policies.

If you've seen one prescription drug monitoring program, you've seen one prescription drug monitoring program. Some are designed well and are easily accessible. Others are frustrating for clinicians and others to use. Some update in real time, while others may have delays of several weeks. Some focus on identifying high-risk patients; others assess prescribers and provide a birds-eye view of prescribing in a community.

One survey found that nearly 3 in 4 physicians reported that access to a prescription drug monitoring program reduced the amount of opioids they prescribed.[9] However, multiple studies have found barriers to prescriber checking of the database, including not being aware of its existence and having problems accessing the information online. Some states have mandated prescriber and pharmacy enrollment in prescription drug monitoring programs, and some even mandate its use prior to prescribing opioids in common clinical situations.[10]

It is not surprising that the outcome data are mixed.[11] Communities can work with their state governments to get the most out of their prescription drug monitoring program, including by helping clinicians connect patients to treatment.

What are take-back days?

Take-back days are publicized occasions for people to return unused opioids and other medications—instead of leaving them at home and at risk for theft and misuse. In November 2017, for example, more than 5,300 sites collected more than 450 tons of "expired, unused, and unwanted" prescription drugs across the country.[12]

The quantity of drugs collected on take-back days is a very tiny fraction of what is dispensed.[13] Their value is mainly in their public message to get rid of extra medications—which is possible for people to do every day. Alternatives to take-back days include mixing up medications with coffee grounds (so they are hard to reclaim later) and throwing the mixture out in the trash or even just flushing unused opioid medications down the toilet. The FDA has developed a "flush list" of medications. This list includes pharmaceuticals where the benefits of toilet disposal far outweigh any environmental risks.[14]

What can the US Food and Drug Administration do to prevent opioid addiction?

The FDA has substantial authority over prescription medications, from approving drug applications to withdrawing drugs from the market—and quite a lot in between. Here are some of the steps the agency can take to support community efforts to address the opioid epidemic.

Closely monitor the marketing of opioids

In the 2000s, the agency was slow to recognize that companies such as Purdue were misleading people about the benefits and risks of opioids. With so much money at stake, these practices have persisted, with officials from another manufacturer of opioids recently pleading guilty to inappropriate sales tactics.[15]

Change the labels of opioid medications

As of 2018, the label on opioid medications does not inform physicians that major reviews have not found evidence of effectiveness of long-term opioid use for chronic pain,[16] with the Centers for Disease Control and Prevention (CDC) finding that "no study of opioid therapy versus placebo, no opioid therapy, or nonopioid therapy for chronic pain evaluated long-term (≥1 year) outcomes related to pain, function, or quality of life."[17] The FDA should also alert physicians to the best evidence on the amount of opioids needed on a short-term basis in specific situations, such as after a tooth extraction or a minor surgical procedure. In April 2018, the FDA commissioner proposed keeping such standards updated on a regular basis, much as the agency does for the appropriate use of antibiotics for specific types of infections.[18]

Change packaging of opioid products

The FDA can require manufacturers to sell opioids in vials that dispense only certain amounts over time, or dose packs that are limited to just a few days. More physicians might prescribe a "5-day dose pack" if it were readily available than the standard 30-day supply.

Restrict the use of certain medications

To maximize the benefits and minimize the harms of medications, the FDA can impose—and then enforce—additional requirements on manufacturers. In 2011, the FDA asked manufacturers to create a special program for some fentanyl products to promote their safe use. The agency's goal was to assure that physicians only prescribed these highly potent opioids to patients who had developed tolerance and were therefore less likely to overdose. In 2012, the agency required manufacturers of long-acting opioids such as OxyContin® to fund education for physicians on appropriate prescribing for pain, with the educational content to be approved by the FDA.

After creating these oversight programs, FDA can assess whether they are working and, if not, strengthen them. In August 2018, however, researchers at Johns Hopkins University reported that the program to safeguard the use of fentanyl products was not working as intended. Many patients who were not tolerant to opioids were receiving the medications, and some were dying from overdose. Yet the oversight program had yet to review a single physician for inappropriate prescribing.[19] The FDA commissioner responded to the new evidence by stating, "We share the concerns about how these drugs are being used and whether the . . . program is working as intended. . . . We're committed to taking new steps to mitigate risks of misuse, abuse, addiction, overdose, and errors associated with these medicines."[20]

The agency's educational program for long-acting opioids has been criticized for not teaching about alternative treatments for pain; it is now being restructured. The FDA is also requiring manufacturers of short-acting opioids to support educational efforts.

Do "abuse-deterrent" formulation of opioids work?

"Abuse deterrent" formulations of opioids are designed to reduce the risk of misuse. One of the major structural flaws of OxyContin® was how easily it could be crushed and snorted or injected. After OxyContin® was reformulated in 2010 to make it more difficult to misuse, overall sales fell, and, perhaps not entirely coincidentally, heroin use began to rise.

This experience exemplifies both the promise and the peril of "abuse-deterrent" formulations. Where successful, the result might wind up creating more harm to the public health.

Opana® was the brand name of an opioid called oxymorphone, which was first approved by FDA in 2006. In 2012, the manufacturer Endo Pharmaceuticals reformulated the medication to prevent snorting and injecting, even though FDA never allowed the company to use the claim of "abuse deterrent."[21] It turned out the modifications generally prevented snorting, but not injecting. As users switched to injecting, the health consequences skyrocketed. Through injection of Opana®, nearly 200 people in Indiana contracted HIV.[22] In 2017, at FDA's request, Endo Pharmaceuticals withdrew the formulation from the market.

The Opana® debacle exemplified how abuse deterrence is not a simple topic. The agency has issued detailed guidance to manufacturers on testing for abuse deterrence,[23] and experts have cautioned the agency to consider a wide range of factors, including the potential to drive people to illicit opioids, in evaluating future requests for abuse deterrence claims.[24]

What other technologies are under development to prevent misuse of opioid pain medications?

In recent years, a wide range of biomedical and public health scientists and entrepreneurs have started to invent new products to prevent the misuse of opioid medications. These innovations aim to assure that only the intended patient can use the medication prescribed, in the correct amounts, and at the right time. These inventions include new types of pill bottles, which only open for the patient; pills with sensors, which assure that they are taken; time-release bottles, which only make pills available when needed; and chemicals that can be mixed with excess opioids and other controlled medications to turn them into a useless gel before discarding. Some of these ideas are promising, but research has yet to determine whether any of these approaches will be effective at reducing the overall harmful consequences of prescription opioids.

What is the role of marijuana in preventing opioid addiction?

Unclear. There is evidence that some of the chemicals in marijuana can help some patients with pain.[25] Based on this idea, advocates have suggested that greater use of marijuana will mean less use of opioids for pain and, as a result, less opioid addiction and fewer overdoses. Evidence for this theory can be found in research suggesting that in states with more liberal marijuana laws, there are fewer opioid prescriptions in Medicare[26] and Medicaid,[27] as well as fewer opioid overdoses.[28]

If such an effect exists, it is likely to be modest. Early marijuana laws did not prevent Rhode Island, Maine, and Vermont from being hit very hard by the opioid epidemic. After one study attributed a decline in opioid-related deaths in 2015 in Colorado to legalization of marijuana,[29] the deaths rose to record levels over the next 2 years.[30]

There is also some evidence to the contrary. Several studies have found that individuals who use medical marijuana are more likely than others to misuse prescription pain medication and to develop an opioid use disorder.[31,32]

Still others have taken the position that the advocates' theory is half right: Yes, alternative pain treatments can save lives from opioids, but no, the answer is not marijuana. They call instead for greater access to other types of treatments with more experience and evidence behind them, such as acupuncture and physical therapy.[33]

Policies that expand access to marijuana may have benefits, but they also carry risks, including the risk of greater use and addiction in young people.[34] As more evidence emerges, policy decisions should be based on data, not on assumptions or ideology.

Can policies go too far in restricting opioid prescribing?

Yes. Policies that make it more difficult to prescribe opioids to patients risk the unintended consequence of hurting patients who do benefit from the medications and are not suffering from addiction. Opioids do relieve pain, and many patients need these medications to ease their suffering and maintain a level of functioning.

Faced with new barriers to treatment, patients who rely on long-term use of opioids have become increasingly vocal. "If they're cutting him back all the way to this, he's not going to be able to function," the wife of one man with fibromyalgia told the *Frederick News-Post* in Maryland. "We're going to lose the house that we've been in for 20 years. Everything that we worked hard for. I want to yell at the insurance company and say, 'Why don't you go ahead and give me the money for his cremation?' Because with these pain patients, they're cutting them back so bad that they're going to want to kill themselves."[35] Indeed, there are websites that track suicides among patients with pain who have difficulty accessing opioids.[36]

If an essential goal of public policy is to maximize benefits and minimize risks, then it is very important for policies on opioid prescribing to be sensitive to the potential for causing harm. That is one reason why the strongest restrictions on prescribing should apply to new patients and not existing patients who are stable on their opioid medication. It is also why the CDC guidelines on the care of patients with chronic, non-cancer pain do not rule out opioid treatment altogether, instead leaving room for clinical judgment and providing guidance on how to assure that ongoing care is meeting its goals. And it is why the FDA commissioner has described his agency's goal as "to reduce overall exposure to opioids, while preserving access for those patients who will benefit."[37]

How can communities support resilience and create a healthy environment to prevent opioid addiction?

One of the fundamental measures of a community's health is the infant mortality rate—the number of infants who die before their first birthday per 1,000 live births. It's a deceptively simple statistic. That is because the infant mortality rate reflects not only the quality of obstetric care but also the health of parents, the nature of their physical and social environment, the state of their nutrition, and so much more. As a result, according to a federal advisory committee, prevention efforts must engage with the whole of how a society "takes care of its most vulnerable citizens."[38]

So it also is with the opioid overdose rate. The proximate cause may be addiction to prescription opioids or illicit drugs, but the phenomenon has deeper roots. Some call it a disease of despair, resulting from a changing economy and loss of upward mobility. Others point to underfunded and failing school systems. Still others note the association of addiction with adverse childhood experiences, such as physical, sexual, and emotional trauma.[39] All of these factors contribute.

Preventing addiction, therefore, calls for a wide lens. Prevention efforts can work by supporting the resilience of individuals and the safety of communities. Promising efforts span a wide range of initiatives aiming to achieve social and economic progress, across multiple social and economic sectors. These include programs to reduce absenteeism and improve school performance, projects to reduce unemployment, and initiatives to lower the level of homicide, suicide, and intimate partner violence in communities.

There is also some evidence that specific educational programs can reduce drug use. Early childhood programs such as the Good Behavior Game help students behave in class, leading to less antisocial behavior, smoking, and other drug use later in life.[40]

Another example is the Communities That Care model, in which local community boards come together and select specific evidence-based prevention programs to implement. The range of options includes programs aimed at bolstering life skills, improving parenting, enhancing family communication, and promoting educational success. In a randomized trial involving 12 communities, youth in places that implemented Communities That Care reported 37% less binge drinking and 23% less alcohol use and were 32% less likely to start using alcohol.[41] Communities interested in implementing this model can contact the Centers for Communities That Care at the University of Washington.[42] Those interested in finding specific programs that might work in their own communities can consult the evidence-based practices web guide of the Substance Abuse and Mental Health Services Administration.[43]

A final consideration for prevention are the roles that tobacco and, to a greater extent, alcohol and marijuana play in adolescence. A common path to opioids starts with these more readily available but addictive substances. Heroin may be the final destination, but it is rarely the first stop. There are effective approaches to preventing youth from smoking, drinking, and using marijuana. These include communication campaigns, targeted taxes that raise prices, enforcement on retailers and other policies that reduce availability to youth. Indirectly, these are policies that counter the opioid epidemic, too.

13

TREATMENT AND RECOVERY POLICY FOR THE OPIOID EPIDEMIC

How important is broad access to effective treatment for opioid addiction?

Top of the list. Treatment does more than just help save individuals one at a time. If treatment is broadly accessible and well-organized into a system of care, then it can bend the curve of the epidemic.

Effective treatment for opioid addiction addresses problems caused by both prescription medications and illicit drugs. The results include fewer overdoses, less crime, smaller drug markets, and more employment—all changes that facilitate economic development. In 2002, the City of Baltimore released the results of a study of about 1,000 people receiving drug and alcohol treatment in 16 programs. The study found a 69% reduction in heroin use and a 64% reduction in illegal activities that persisted a year after the initiation of treatment, as well as major improvements in employment and reductions in the use of cocaine and alcohol.[1]

Effective treatment also works as prevention. That's because, in its own way, opioid addiction is a contagious disease. Someone who is misusing opioids can sell or share them with their friends and neighbors; that same person in treatment, however, can help others stay away from trouble or connect to services. More people in treatment means fewer opportunities for young people to come across opioids to misuse and, perhaps most important, more people at home helping them succeed at school and at work.

What are the elements of a robust treatment system?

A successful treatment *program* offers high quality services to a group of patients. A robust treatment *system* offers the full range of effective services to a population. These services should be based on evidence of what works, offered at sufficient scale, be well coordinated, and of high quality.

What works

Three important elements of an effective treatment system for opioid addiction are access to medications, counseling and other health services in multiple settings, and a variety of supports.

The three Food and Drug Administration (FDA) approved medications for opioid addiction are methadone, buprenorphine, and naltrexone. There is significant evidence, especially for methadone and buprenorphine, that medication use increases retention in treatment, reduces the risk for overdose, and helps people to achieve remission and recovery. As the Department of Health and Human Services recently stated, "ongoing medication treatment for [opioid use disorder] is linked to better retention and outcomes than treatment without medications."[2] The use of medications is backed by the National Institutes of Health,[3] the Centers for Disease Control and Prevention,[4] and the World Health Organization,[5] among other leading scientific authorities.

Most people respond well to treatment in community settings, such as primary care or a local opioid treatment program. A therapeutic environment such as a residential treatment center can also be helpful at the start of treatment for people with severe opioid use disorder, particularly when complicated by addiction to other substances and significant social needs. Regardless of the setting, individuals should have access to counseling (to address triggers for opioid misuse), other health services (including mental health and medical care), and support for recovery (to help patients put their lives back together).

Sufficient scale

One small treatment program is not enough for a community confronting the opioid epidemic. Scale means not only enough treatment for all in need but ready access as well. There should not be waiting lists. People should be able to start treatment on the same day they walk in the door.

Well coordinated

Treatment settings should be well connected to one another. There should be an open front door that can start effective therapy quickly (such as in the emergency department or through mobile outreach) and a strong effort to transition people to ongoing, effective care.

In the mid-2000s, the City of Baltimore launched the Baltimore Buprenorphine Initiative. This program provided rapid access to treatment that included buprenorphine and counseling in 6 treatment centers across the city. Once patients were stabilized, the programs transferred their care to community health centers and other primary care practices. Each patient was assigned an outreach worker to assure the transition was effective and to connect the patient to social services as needed. The initiative helped Baltimore reduce heroin overdose deaths by 75% from 1999 to 2010, with about half of the decline attributed to the increased access to buprenorphine.[6]

European countries have developed extensive systems of care for opioid addiction. Countries such as France,[7] Spain, and Portugal have seen major reductions in overdose and other complications of addiction alongside increases in access to treatment that includes methadone and buprenorphine. These countries also have extensive services available to people with opioid addiction who are not at the moment interested in treatment.

Here's a case example. In Barcelona, Spain, a 45-year-old man who uses heroin shows up at a drop-in center, saying he is having trouble finding heroin to purchase that day. He obtains a dose of methadone from the addiction medicine physician who works there. The next day, he returns for another dose of methadone and engages with a social worker and psychologist about what's going on in his life. Over the next few weeks, he develops enough trust to attend a formal drug treatment program. It's located upstairs.

High quality

A final characteristic of effective treatment systems is ongoing quality assessment. Outpatient treatment programs are regulated by state agencies and the federal government, as well as by private accreditors. Community leaders can track the key metrics of quality and service for the programs in their areas. Ideally, this oversight should be focused not just on specific regulatory requirements (such as the security of controlled substances) but also on public health outcomes (such as progress in treatment and reduction in overdoses).

Should hospital emergency departments start treatment for opioid addiction?

Yes. When Willie Sutton was asked why he robbed banks, he famously replied, "Because that's where the money is." Why should emergency departments start addiction treatment? Because that's where the patients are.

Patients with opioid addiction come to the emergency department after overdosing. They also come with injuries, flare-ups of other chronic illnesses such as diabetes and heart failure, and acute conditions such as asthma attacks. They even come with complaints of pain in the hope of receiving opioids to misuse. Every emergency department visit is an opportunity to provide access to addiction treatment.

Typically, emergency departments give out phone numbers or, in extraordinary circumstances, make appointments for people in addiction treatment centers. Evidence is emerging, however, that referrals are not enough. By starting people on treatment medication right away, emergency departments can save lives.

Here's why: People with untreated opioid addiction in the emergency department are just a few hours away from experiencing severe withdrawal symptoms. If a nurse or social worker sends someone home with a phone number for a treatment program, it's very likely that the person will use 2 or 3 times before being able to call the next morning. By then, the moment for change may have passed.

A better approach: the emergency department can provide a dose of buprenorphine plus a referral to care the next day. The dose prevents withdrawal and gives people a chance to follow through. In a randomized study, offering buprenorphine in the emergency department more than doubled the rate of continued treatment with a primary care physician 1 month later.[8]

Where else should people with opioid addiction be able to start treatment?

Primary care

After completing an 8-hour training course, primary care clinicians can prescribe buprenorphine for addiction treatment. They can also prescribe injectable depot naltrexone, another FDA-approved medication. And they can collaborate with local opioid treatment programs to provide quick access to methadone.

Unfortunately, far too few primary doctors offer addiction treatment. Fewer than 5% of physicians have obtained the required training to prescribe buprenorphine,[9] and there are substantial disparities between regions.[10] Areas where few physicians are trained also tend to have few specialty addiction treatment providers. As a result, there is limited access to care in large swaths of the country.

Jails and prisons

Instead of forcing patients to go through withdrawal after an arrest, the correctional system can start treatment. The American Correctional Association has joined with the American Society of Addiction Medicine to call for expansions in treatment in detention.[11] Recently, Rhode Island reported what happened after the state expanded access to treatment for all inmates in jail and prison with all 3 FDA-approved medications and made connections for ongoing care in the community: fatal overdoses among those leaving jail and prison dropped by 60%.[12]

Outreach sites

A recent development is mobile treatment.[13] Clinical teams start treatment in syringe services programs, shelters for individuals who are homeless, and other community locations.

Do gaps in payment and insurance coverage limit access to opioid addiction treatment?

Yes. Many people who desperately need addiction treatment cannot afford care. Of 10 Americans addicted to opioids, alcohol, marijuana, and other substances, 9 fail to receive care each year, with many pointing to a lack of a source of payment as an explanation.[14] There are major gaps in coverage offered by both public programs and private insurance companies for addiction treatment. These gaps are a major reason why robust treatment systems are rarely found in the United States.

Public programs

Medicaid, Medicare, other public grant-funded programs and the correctional system all pay for addiction treatment, but none consistently offers access to all evidence-based services.

With 73 million Americans covered,[15] Medicaid is the largest payer of addiction treatment in the country. It is especially important in the 37 states (as of November 26, 2018) that have adopted some form of Medicaid expansion under the Affordable Care Act.[16] That is because the expansion adds low-income, single adults to coverage. It has been estimated that a million people newly insured by Medicaid have mental health disorders or addiction.[17]

Medicaid expansion does not guarantee coverage of all opioid addiction treatment options, however. The list of services that are paid for varies considerably state to state, with only 13 Medicaid programs in 2018 covering all services recommended by the American Society of Addiction Medicine.[18] Some states do not cover methadone at all; many impose preauthorization and other restrictions on treatment with buprenorphine. States vary widely in providing access to even short-term residential treatment.[19] And even when states do cover addiction treatment, low reimbursement rates can dissuade high-quality providers from participating.

Medicare, the nation's public insurance program for older adults, covers outpatient counseling from licensed practitioners as well as the medications buprenorphine and depot naltrexone through Medicare Part D. In 2018, Congress passed legislation authorizing Medicare coverage of treatment with methadone for the first time. Medicare, however, does not cover residential treatment.

Since 2016, Congress has provided considerable extra funding for treatment outside of the Medicaid and Medicare programs. Much of this funding has gone to states in the form of grants. This funding has made treatment services more widely available in many areas. However, it is unclear for how long the federal government will make this supplemental funding available. This uncertainly limits the ability of treatment providers to invest in a durable expansion of services.

Jails and prisons can offer addiction treatment. However, it is the rare jail or prison that offers a full-range of services backed by evidence. In most jails across the country, individuals with an opioid addiction are forced to endure painful (and occasionally fatal[20]) withdrawal. Even when the court system provides access to treatment, in the vast majority of cases, the treatment does not include the medications most likely to be successful.[21]

Private insurers

A majority of Americans with health insurance have private coverage. Yet private insurance does not have a stellar record of providing access to a full range of effective addiction treatment services. Congress passed the Mental Health Parity and Addiction Equity Act to fix this problem. Under this law—in theory—private insurers are prohibited from offering less coverage for addiction than offered for medical illnesses such as diabetes. However—in practice—insurers rarely cover care in opioid treatment programs that offer methadone and impose a variety of other limitations on addiction treatment. Attorneys General in some states have filed suit under the parity law in an attempt to force greater access to care.[22]

What happens when the treatment system falls short in providing access to effective care?

In areas without sufficient Medicaid reimbursement, state funding, or other insurer coverage, clinics pop up that offer services, including access to methadone and buprenorphine, for cash. Communities are often frustrated with the rapid appearance and disappearance of such clinics, with local experts often noting concerns with the quality of care. Sometimes news reports mistakenly blame these problems on the medications themselves,[23] when, in fact, the existence of these clinics is a symptom of insufficient insurance coverage for high-quality care.

There are also many short- and long-term residential programs that do a brisk cash business. Some are expensive programs for well-off individuals with costs that can exceed $30,000 per month. Others follow the Florida model, which *The New York Times* defines as "counseling during the day—usually chair-circles of group therapy—in what is typically a residential building" and living in a "sober living home" by night."[24] The Florida model typically costs about $9,000 a month.

Low-quality residential programs aggressively seek out patients, advertising on television and paying recruiters finders' fees.[25] Some insurers will cover a brief stay at these residential programs. When the benefits run out, the programs demand that families pay tens of thousands of dollars to continue treatment. Many of these programs offer little more than pep talks and admonitions not to use drugs; others offer dangerous, unproven treatments that pose significant risks.[26] Relapse rates can be very high.[27]

The popularity of expensive residential programs reflects the predatory behavior of treatment entrepreneurs—as well as the desperation of families who live in areas without robust treatment systems.

Why are there so few robust treatment systems for opioid addiction in the United States?

Given the strong evidence that addiction treatment is a critical part of the solution to the opioid epidemic, it is natural to wonder: Why is there such poor access to care? A major reason is inadequate coverage, both by public programs and by private insurers. Two other factors are regulatory barriers and stigma.

The two medications most supported by evidence—methadone and buprenorphine—are subject to significant federal and state regulation. Under federal law, which dates back to the Nixon Administration, methadone may only be provided for addiction treatment in licensed "opioid treatment programs." These are specifically designated centers subject to a host of regulations that specify how the medication can be distributed and what services must be offered to individuals receiving care.

On top of federal rules, some states have set their own limits on methadone access. Despite having the highest rate of death from drug overdoses in the country, West Virginia has long had a moratorium in place on new locations for opioid treatment programs statewide.

Buprenorphine faces a different set of regulatory standards. Only physicians who complete an 8-hour training program can prescribe the medication for addiction, and there are limits on the number of patients that such physicians can care for at once. Several states, including Tennessee and West Virginia, have added their own state regulations on buprenorphine treatment. These rules require extensive documentation and the provision of additional services to patients, regardless of whether these are needed. Federal law permits nurse practitioners and physician assistants to prescribe buprenorphine after even more extensive training, but not all states allow them to do so.

Are all these regulations really needed? No. European countries do not subject treatment medications to such extensive regulation. Many people are able to access addiction care in drop-in centers, pharmacies, physician offices, and treatment centers.

Meanwhile, back in the United States, physicians are allowed to prescribe opioids without these special restrictions—but only to treat pain, not when the purpose is treating addiction. In other words, the U.S. system makes it easier for doctors to cause addiction than to treat it. The origin of this paradox can be found in history; since the Harrison Act of 1914, laws in the United States have reflected deep skepticism and stigma about long-term treatment of people with addiction. This stigma on treatment persists to the present day. Many health-care providers refuse to offer addiction treatment, saying it is "not my job." Ask them whose job it is, and they may point to 12-step programs, specialty addiction providers—or even the police. As a result, in many communities, there is little effort by physician practices, emergency departments, and hospitals to offer treatment services, even in locations devastated by the opioid epidemic that have virtually no other potential sources of care.

Complicating the situation is the myth that treatment with methadone or buprenorphine is "addiction by another means." This myth is quite persistent, reinforced by politicians, news-paper editors, and even individuals in recovery. It can be fostered by advocates of residential programs with an ideolog-ical aversion to medications as well as by friends and family of those with addiction who do not like the idea of their loved one taking a medication, least of all an opioid.

These barriers all reinforce each other. Inadequate payment and insurance coverage, overregulation of treatment, histor-ical reluctance to provide care in the healthcare system, and the stigma on medications all come together to limit access to life-saving care.

What is "not in my backyard" syndrome?

"Not in my backyard" syndrome is "a colloquialism signifying one's opposition to the locating of something considered unde-sirable in one's neighborhood."[28] The term—and its shorthand version, NIMBY—emerged to describe public objections to the siting of toxic waste facilities, incinerators, and nuclear power plants. But some communities oppose the existence of addic-tion treatment programs as if they too were environmental hazards, reflecting the tremendous stigma that still exists.

When news surfaces that a new addiction treatment pro-gram is opening in an area, neighbors often fear a decline in property values; the arrival of undesirable people from other parts of a city, county, or state; the greater use of alcohol and drugs; and increases in crime. A common complaint is that some communities have more than their "fair share" of human service programs (such as public housing, clinics for individuals with mental illness, and services for individuals and families experiencing homelessness). The NIMBY syndrome leads residents to call on local political leaders to enact zoning and other restrictions to keep addiction treatment programs away.

Community opposition to addiction treatment can have several harmful consequences. First, and most obviously, it can block the establishment of needed services. Second, as the US Department of Health and Human Services (HHS) has noted, "even if a program ultimately prevails, the fight can be costly, not only in terms of resources, but in its effects on the clients as well."[29] Third, the NIMBY syndrome reinforces the stigma on addiction, making it more difficult for individuals and families to confront their problems and seek assistance.

Addressing NIMBY is critical to the successful expansion of effective addiction treatment programs in communities across the country. There are several key steps to doing so.

Address fears with evidence

Many people who fear the opening of a treatment program do not understand the nature of opioid addiction or its responsiveness to treatment. Constructive engagement that involves people in recovery alongside treatment experts can help dispel these myths.

It is also important to share the considerable evidence that addiction treatment programs do not cause crime or other adverse effects. HHS has found,

> In almost every instance, a community's fear of having an alcohol or other drug treatment program located within its borders is unfounded. In reality, treatment

programs pose no legitimate danger to the health or welfare of the residents, nor do they draw substance abusers and pushers to the area. In fact, alcohol and other drug treatment programs improve neighborhoods by helping people get well.[30]

For a recent study in Baltimore, researchers went to extraordinary lengths to evaluate the impact of addiction treatment programs on violent crime.[31] They mapped each block of the city, noting the locations of different types of businesses, from corner stores to drug treatment programs. The study found that corner stores, liquor stores, and convenience stores had far greater association with violence than drug treatment programs. Because effective treatment for opioid addiction reduces criminal behavior, the net result of more drug treatment over the long term is very positive for communities.

Engaging the media can also be helpful. When an elected official in Baltimore criticized addiction treatment programs, *The Baltimore Sun* was quick to respond. "She says she believes treatment centers 'tear neighborhoods and communities apart,'" wrote the editors. "In fact, it is addiction that tears neighborhoods and communities apart, and we need to address the problem where it exists."[32]

Be prepared to litigate

Laws that forbid discrimination against treatment programs include the Americans with Disabilities Act, the Fair Housing Act, the equal protection clause of the 14th Amendment to the Constitution as well as other state and local statutes. Of these, the most useful may be the Americans with Disabilities Act, which states, "No qualified individual with a disability shall, by reason of such disability, be excluded from participation in or be denied the benefits of the services, programs, or activities of a public entity, or be subjected to discrimination by any such entity."[33] Many successful challenges to NIMBY protests have cited these words.

Be a good neighbor

Once established, treatment programs should act like constructive members of a community, contributing to local activities and participating in community events. There should be pathways for community members to ask questions and protocols to reduce the chance of disturbances. Many communities find common ground through the creation of "good neighbor" agreements. Regular opportunities for tours can help people understand that the program is a place where people go to regain control over their lives. HHS explains,

> Once a treatment program has opened its facility, the battle is not over. Fences must be continually tended and repaired. Studies show that communities that opposed treatment programs generally become more accepting over time, as they see the benefits that the programs bring. However, neglecting community relations, even for a short time, can open old rifts or create new ones that make future operations or expansion difficult.[34]

Why is there resistance in some minority communities to addiction treatment programs?

Opposition in some minority communities to addiction treatment programs is more complicated than the NIMBY syndrome. As Columbia historian Samuel Kelton Roberts Jr. has noted, the introduction of treatment programs, including those that provided methadone, was perceived by some as an intrusion by predominantly white institutions into minority communities. There was much less financial support for locally run treatment centers that would have concurrently offered access to a variety of social services. Today, treatment programs run by outside entities or private companies can be perceived as profiting from the suffering of a community. Understanding this history, hiring from within a community and engaging in candid dialogue are important steps to bridging these gaps.

Can treatment expansions backfire?

Well-executed expansions of treatment have predictably positive effects on individuals and communities. However, poorly designed treatment expansions may actually worsen the epidemic. Three common mistakes are investing in the wrong services, ignoring community concerns, and failing to assure a high quality of care.

Investing in the wrong services

Some communities direct new funding to "detox" programs. However, what people call "detox" is not addiction treatment; it's just a few days of care to reduce the symptoms associated with withdrawal. People who go through "detox" often continue to intensely crave opioids and, having lost tolerance, are at high risk for overdose when their use resumes.

Other communities seek to expand short-term, residential programs that do not allow people to receive FDA-approved medications for opioid addiction. These programs may have strong support from local advocates and individuals who have graduated and credit the treatment programs and their philosophies with their success. But many also contribute to the overdose problem.

In Kentucky, for example, the centerpiece of the state's investment in treatment was a network of 15 programs known as "Recovery Kentucky." Thousands of individuals received services in these programs each year. Yet the programs were largely based on a "drug-free" model with roots in the 12-step treatment for alcohol addiction. As journalist Jason Cherkis documented in his Pulitzer Prize–nominated report, "Dying to Be Free,"[35] most of the programs were averse to allowing individuals to receive effective medications. In fact, some even counseled that taking medications precluded true recovery. "It's being alive," one program supervisor told Cherkis. "But you're not clean and sober."

After the state reported a sky-high success rate for Recovery Kentucky, Cherkis dug deeper. The statistics didn't include those who dropped out, which could include as many as 3 in 4 of those who participated. When one director of a large treatment program was asked about the experience of graduates of her program, she responded, "How would I have that?" Only when patients relapsed and returned did the programs know what had happened. Cherkis noted, "For the treatment centers, the revolving door can be financially lucrative."

While Kentucky has expanded access to treatment with medications since the time of Cherkis's report, major barriers to care still exist. Kentucky had 1,419 overdose deaths in 2016, the fifth highest rate in the nation.[36] The opioid overdose rate increased by 12% from the prior year.[37]

Ignoring community concerns

A typical story is that an effective addiction treatment program becomes a victim of its own success. It might have opened at a time of tremendous stress, drug use, and crime. Gradually, as more individuals obtain treatment, crime in the area declines and property values rise. New neighbors may then become upset at the presence of the treatment program. Where the NIMBY syndrome kicks into high gear, the new neighbors can harass the clients and staff of the treatment program and encourage elected officials to try to shut it down. "To the patients, it's ironic," one observer of opposition to an opioid treatment program in Brooklyn noted. "At a time when they have chosen to turn their lives around, become productive members of society, they are frowned upon as 'the problem.'"[38]

To avoid setbacks in access to care, public officials and treatment programs should actively address community concerns, while continuing to explain the value of treatment to new groups of residents.

Poor-quality care

Rapid expansions in access to treatment require rapid shifts in funding, which may entice inexperienced or unqualified operators of treatment programs into areas. Poorly run treatment programs not only may have low success rates, but they can also fuel misunderstanding about treatment and spark community opposition. Communities should support responsible oversight of clinics by state and federal agencies, with transparency about programmatic challenges and plans to address them.

How can a robust treatment system support pregnant women with opioid addiction?

Women with opioid addiction need access to effective treatment before, during, and after a pregnancy. Robust systems of care can offer nurse-led home visiting programs to help with a myriad of challenges facing new families. States and localities can also support specific clinical models to help parents and children thrive, such as the Drug Free Moms and Babies Program in West Virginia, which offers robust and ongoing counseling, coaching, services, and care to families after delivery.[39] Comprehensive programs that utilize medications for addiction treatment have led to more successful family outcomes, including less need for out-of-home foster care placement.[40]

Not as helpful is a narrow focus on caring for babies who have neonatal abstinence syndrome, known as NAS. NAS refers to the short-term withdrawal symptoms that babies experience after birth, which are treatable with a few days to a couple of weeks of medication. NAS itself represents only a small risk for a newborn compared to the major threat of a parent with untreated addiction. Newborn nurseries that take care of babies with NAS should do more than monitor their treatment protocols. They should establish relationships with addiction treatment programs to help support parents and adopt outcome metrics related to parental health.

What is the controversy over forcing people with opioid addiction into treatment?

When an individual with mental illness is suicidal or a threat to others, physicians have the authority to hold them in a hospital for their own protection. After a few days, if the risk to self or others is still high, the physicians can ask a judge to extend the period of treatment behind locked doors. This process is called civil commitment.

As the opioid epidemic has grown, some parents of young people with addiction have begun to call for expanding the use of civil commitment. Several states have laws that permit people with addiction to be held against their will and ordered into treatment, even if they have not committed a crime. Massachusetts is the state that has used this power most frequently. The state has sent thousands of individuals against their will to receive treatment. However, the treatment available has rarely included access to FDA-approved medications, with reports of mistreatment and abuse leading to a lawsuit from the American Civil Liberties Union.[41] In 2018, a proposal by the Massachusetts governor that would have expanded civil commitment to allow emergency department physicians to hold patients with opioid addiction for 3 days against their will did not pass the state's general assembly.[42]

There is no justification for forcing people with opioid addiction into substandard treatment. However, there is controversy about whether civil commitment to effective treatment might ever make sense. Some argue that the act of forcing people into treatment makes it less likely treatment will be successful; people may not take medications given to them or they may sit in a counseling session but not really listen. Others believe that holding someone against his or her will is a violation of fundamental civil liberties. There are many caregivers and others, however, who see a few days of civil commitment coupled with effective treatment as an opportunity to help people whose brains are not functioning normally make it through a particularly dangerous window of time. This debate is likely to remain intense for some time.

What is the role of communities in supporting people in treatment and recovery?

Communities should assess whether their local policies are complicating the ability of people with opioid addiction to achieve a full recovery. Many housing, job training, and educational programs unnecessarily exclude people with a history of addiction, such as those arrested for non-violent drug offenses. These exclusions reduce the opportunities available to people for turning their lives around. Communities can change such practices. Other promising steps include:

Offering peer support

Individuals in treatment face a host of personal and social challenges poorly understood by those who have not walked in their shoes. That is why many treatment programs employ peers to provide support and assistance.[43] It is also why peer-led drop-in centers are popular at all hours of the night, when cravings might otherwise trigger people to relapse.[44] Communities can support peer programs by providing training and credentialing and by advocating for insurance reimbursement. In Rhode Island, every hospital is required to employ peers to engage with people who have experienced an overdose.

Expanding housing assistance

Many people with severe addiction experience homelessness. This condition is not only physically dangerous and emotionally traumatic, but it also complicates efforts to receive ongoing treatment for both medical and behavioral health conditions. Housing First models that provide a residence up front (rather than wait for criteria to be met) have been shown to be particularly effective.[45]

Yet, housing options are often lacking for individuals as they start treatment. Their addiction may have led to eviction, even by their own families, even from their own homes. Prior convictions may make it impossible for them to qualify for federal and state public housing programs. Poorly regulated "recovery homes" may not offer a stable environment.

Another approach is for communities to offer "supportive housing"—residences for individuals where they can also receive mental health and other services. For individuals with severe addiction to alcohol, for example, such programs have been associated with fewer emergency department visits and arrests and declines in public expenditures overall.[46] While Medicaid cannot pay for the costs of housing, the program can fund the services to individuals who live there.

Establishing employment programs

Many individuals with addiction are unemployed and have trouble finding and keeping jobs. Yet stable employment, and the income it generates, can help individuals reconnect with their families and develop productive routines that do not involve drug use. Promising programs, based on models developed for people with mental illness, provide specific employment training and opportunities for people in recovery.[47]

14

HARM REDUCTION POLICY FOR THE OPIOID EPIDEMIC

What Is harm reduction?

Harm reduction is "a set of practical strategies aimed at reducing negative consequences associated with drug use." It is also "a movement for social justice built on a belief in, and respect for, the rights of people who use drugs." These two concepts—as explained by the Harm Reduction Coalition[1]—may appear to be quite different but, in fact, are inseparable. That's because it is often a lack of "respect for the rights of people who use drugs" that blocks efforts to address the "negative consequences associated with drug use."[2]

Harm reduction starts with the principle that the lives of people who use drugs are worth saving. From this vantage point, access to addiction treatment is a harm reduction strategy. So too is the provision of essential social services. Harm reduction also includes a variety of programs to help the many users who are not currently interested in treatment. These programs keep people alive, help them protect and care for themselves, and begin a process of engagement that can lead to effective treatment and recovery.

A key principle of harm reduction is listening to people who use drugs for their perspective on the dangers they face. For example, users might explain that a treatment program has not been successful in helping users because staff there belittle participants. Users also can provide input in the design of services so that they do not reinforce unpleasant or traumatic experiences.

Harm reduction also recognizes the social context of drug use—including the "realities of poverty, class, racism, social isolation, past trauma, sex-based discrimination and other social inequalities."[3] As a result, effective harm reduction approaches not only provide specific services but also aim to support users of drugs with the major challenges in their lives.

Examples of effective harm reduction programs include:

- distribution of the reversal medication naloxone, to support reversal of overdoses in the community;
- syringe services, to provide clean needles and other materials to reduce the risk of infectious disease transmission;
- drug checking, to inform individuals about the contents of illicit substances; and
- overdose prevention sites, to provide a safer environment for drug use that includes access to immediate resuscitation, as well as treatment opportunities.

Not everyone who advocates for people who use drugs supports every harm reduction effort. For example, some consider drug addiction as a matter of individual autonomy, rather than as a loss of control, and may object to offering treatment inside naloxone and syringe services programs as paternalistic.

Moreover, not every program with the label of "harm reduction" is successful in reaching its goals. This is why the field is committed to research and evaluation and to making changes in response to information about what is working and what is not. Because of this focus on outcomes, its respect for individuals, and its engagement

with communities, harm reduction is fundamentally a
public health strategy.

What are naloxone distribution programs?

Naloxone distribution programs aim to make this medication available to individuals most likely to be in a position to
save lives from overdose. To succeed, these programs must
distribute naloxone much further and wider than would
be possible with the traditional requirement of individual
prescriptions for each patient.

One of the first naloxone programs started in 1996 in
Chicago, where a mobile program distributed naloxone to
more than 10,000 people over the next decade. Participants reported more than 1,000 reported overdose reversals.[4] By 2010,
a national survey found that more than 175 naloxone programs
in 15 states had reported more than 10,000 reversals.[5] The recent surge in overdose deaths has caused a major expansion
of naloxone distribution programs around the country—with
particular interest by state and local law enforcement agencies.
Hundreds of police departments are now equipping and
training their officers in naloxone use.

Naloxone distribution programs may require a change
in state law to permit individuals who have not themselves
seen a physician to acquire the medication. In North Carolina,
Maryland, New York, and elsewhere, the law permits public
health officials to issue standing orders for naloxone for an entire community, so that anyone can go to a pharmacy to receive
a dose to have at the ready in case of a witnessed overdose.
More than 1,400 pharmacies in North Carolina now participate
in the program.[6]

Well-designed research studies have shown that naloxone distribution programs save lives. For example,
one study compared communities in Massachusetts that
implemented naloxone programs with those that did not.

This research found that the two sets of communities were similar in many ways, including the number of non-fatal overdoses. But those with naloxone distribution programs experienced significantly lower opioid-related deaths. The researchers concluded that the study provided evidence that naloxone distribution programs are "an effective public health intervention to address increasing mortality in the opioid overdose epidemic by training potential bystanders to prevent, recognize, and respond to opioid overdoses."[7]

What is the case for making naloxone available without a prescription?

Similar to how cardiac defibrillators halt dangerous disturbances in heart rhythms, naloxone reverses overdoses and saves lives. The more broadly available, the more lives naloxone can save.

There are two ways to make naloxone more accessible. One approach is already in effect in more than a dozen states: a local health officer or physician provides a standing order, allowing anyone in a community to go to the pharmacy to get a dose. This approach encourages pharmacists to provide some basic training to individuals. However, it is dependent on whether local laws permit this arrangement and whether there's a physician willing to write the standing order.

An even better solution would be for naloxone to be available over-the-counter. The Food and Drug Administration (FDA) has the authority to allow such sales, but only after evidence is presented to the agency that consumers can use the product successfully without the engagement of a health professional. The FDA is now providing guidance to manufacturers to assist with gathering such evidence.[8] If successful, an over-the-counter switch would provide much greater access to naloxone across the country. If this happens, insurers should pay for over-the-counter naloxone just as they do for prescribed naloxone.

Otherwise, a switch to over-the-counter status might actually reduce access to this life-saving medication.

What are good samaritan laws?

Even if naloxone has already been administered and the overdose has been reversed, people on the scene should call 911 for an ambulance. That is because the effects of naloxone wear off quickly, while the underlying opioid may persist in the user's body and cause a second and possibly fatal overdose. Unfortunately, many contacts of people who use drugs are afraid that if they call 911, the police will respond to the scene of a drug overdose and charge them with a crime.

To address this fear, as of July 2017, 38 US states have a good samaritan statute in place.[9] These laws prohibit the police from leveling low-level charges such as possession of controlled substances against people who call 911. Good samaritan laws, however, do not protect callers against more serious charges, such as drug trafficking or driving while under the influence.

In some states, good samaritan laws condition the legal protection on specific actions, such as waiting for first responders to arrive. In a few states, the laws only allow for "assisting an overdose victim" to be a mitigating factor at sentencing.[10] In general, the broader the immunity, the more likely someone is to call 911. It is also critical for there to be broad awareness of the protections, both among law enforcement officers and the public. When high-risk users of opioids in Washington State learned of the good samaritan law there, 88% reported a greater likelihood to call 911.[11]

What are syringe services programs?

Syringe services programs offer clean needles and other supplies, as well as training on safer drug use, to users of intravenous drugs across the United States. The programs developed as a response to the HIV/AIDS crisis in the 1980s, after it was recognized that the virus was moving from person to person through the sharing of needles.

From the outset, syringe services programs were controversial, with some claiming that the programs were encouraging illicit activity. In the years and decades since, these concerns have been thoroughly addressed by research. Numerous studies have found that these programs do not increase the amount of drug use or reduce interest in treatment.[12]

One fascinating study assessed what happened when Windham, Connecticut, shut down its syringe services program as a result of community opposition. Researchers interviewed more than 100 former users of the site and collected data on discarded syringes and bags of illicit drugs. They found major increases in syringe sharing as well as "significant increases . . . in the percentage of respondents who reported an unreliable source as their source of syringes." The researchers also found that the number of syringes found in parks and streets increased.[13]

Beyond reducing the spread of infectious disease, syringe services programs offer a number of important benefits. These include reducing the number of syringes found in public areas[14,15] and lowering the risk of needle stick injury to police and other first responders.[16] Programs also can connect people to social services such as housing, food assistance, and job training.

And, in an especially promising trend, some syringe services programs have started offering initial doses of buprenorphine to individuals ready to start treatment. In June 2018, for example, the city of Burlington, Vermont, announced that the state's largest syringe program would offer buprenorphine prescriptions on site. "We really need to meet these clients where they are and make treatment as easily available to them as possible," said one of the program's coordinators. "We find the hardest thing for people is that first step. It's making that first step easier."[17]

What are the controversies over how syringe services programs are managed?

One operational question for syringe services programs is how many syringes to distribute to each client at each session. Some programs set a cap at 10 or 20 and require a 1:1 exchange, on the grounds that these steps minimize the chance that syringes will be discarded in the community.

Such rules, however, may undermine the effectiveness of the syringe program. Requiring a 1:1 exchange may mean that people receive fewer clean syringes than they really need, leading to syringe sharing and all of the problems that the programs are intended to avoid.[18] Of course, on the other extreme, giving out too many syringes at a time can create a secondary market and reduce the number of interactions that the program has with clients—interactions that can lead to treatment, housing, and connection to other services.

The most successful programs (a) encourage syringe return without requiring a 1:1 match and (b) aim to distribute the right number of syringes for short-term personal use, creating opportunities for repeat visits and engagement.

A second operational question is the role of single-use syringes. These syringes allow for one fill; their needles automatically retract after the plunger is pushed all the way in. However, it is still possible for these syringes to be shared: Users can pass around the syringe and split the single dose before it is exhausted.

Some communities have adopted policies requiring their syringe services program to use single-use syringes, on the theory that this will reduce the risk of needle sticks in the community. However, a policy of exclusively distributing single-use syringes may backfire. Here's why: If 2 people are each given 5 single-use syringes, they have an incentive to share so that each can use opioids 10 times. (If they do not share, each will be able to use opioids just 5 times.)

Exclusively distributing an inadequate number of single-use syringes not only risks more sharing but also could create an underground market for regular syringes, which may then be discarded and pose risks to the community.

What is drug checking?

Drug checking is a service that provides information to people about what is in their street drugs. It is particularly relevant to situations where purchasers do not know for sure what they have bought. Originally developed in Europe to test club drugs during "raves," drug checking is emerging as a strategy to combat the fentanyl epidemic.

Drug checking can occur either on site or remotely. On-site testing allows people who use drugs to know right away whether the pills or other illicit materials they have purchased include particularly dangerous substances. Thus forewarned, people may opt not to take the drugs or use a smaller quantity. With remote testing, people submit a tiny sample of drugs and receive a code for anonymous look-up of the results a few days later.

Drug checking offers advantages both to individuals and the community. People who use drugs can take steps to protect themselves and warn others, as part of what Johns Hopkins Professor Susan Sherman has called "consumer protection" in the illicit drug market.[19] Communities benefit by aggregating the results of testing to obtain real-time information on the composition of drugs in their area.

At the same time, however, drug checking carries risks. One major risk is that the results will be wrong and provide a false sense of security to people who use drugs. A second risk is that individuals will use drug checking to seek out the more potent drugs (including fentanyl), potentially shifting the market in a dangerous direction.

Beginning in late 2013, as the ultra-high potency opioid fentanyl began to be mixed with heroin and other illicit substances in the United States, drug users began to die in unprecedented numbers. A major reason is that users were often not aware of what they were buying. Could drug checking help? That was the question asked by Professor Sherman and Brown University researcher Traci Green, who launched a study on fentanyl checking in the United States.[20]

The two researchers tested 3 technologies to see if they could accurately detect fentanyl on site. One of the 3 technologies—a testing strip originally developed to test for the presence of fentanyl in urine—did so reliably. Two other technologies were more difficult to use and less accurate (but provided additional information that might be useful).[21]

The researchers also interviewed more than 300 people who use drugs as well as several dozen people who work in harm reduction organizations, such as syringe services programs. They found that "the vast majority of people who use drugs have a high degree of concern about fentanyl in the drug supply," with more than 4 in 5 people worried that their drugs might contain fentanyl and hopeful that drug checking would help them protect themselves from overdose.[22] Service providers supported fentanyl checking as well, both because of the information it can provide and because it would serve "as a point for greater engagement in services, including syringe service programs and treatment for substance use disorder."[23]

Professors Sherman and Green concluded that "drug checking strategies are reliable, practical, and very much desired by those at greatest risk of overdose." They recommended that "public health and harm reduction agencies . . . implement anonymous drug checking as part of a public health strategy to save lives from fentanyl." Such a strategy, they advised, should link drug checking to harm reduction counseling, health education, and opioid addiction treatment.

Based on this study and other research, a growing number of local organizations and agencies are offering fentanyl test strips along with syringe services, naloxone distribution, access to treatment, and other harm reduction services.

What are overdose prevention sites?

Overdose prevention sites—also called supervised consumption spaces—are sites where individuals can bring their drugs and use them. On-site personnel stand ready to resuscitate those who overdose. After the first site opened in 1986 in Bern, Switzerland, the concept spread to other cities and countries across Europe, including the Netherlands, Germany, Spain, Australia, and Canada.[24]

Some overdose prevention sites are co-located with other services. For example, sites in Spain offer medical care, health education, counseling, and case management, often with an addiction treatment program upstairs or nearby. Other facilities stand alone, offering referrals to nearby services. There are a few mobile units, including in Berlin, Barcelona, and Copenhagen.

In the United States, the idea of a place where people can come to use illicit drugs is politically controversial. In August 2018, the deputy attorney general of the United States did not mince words when he called a supervised consumption facility a "taxpayer-sponsored haven to shoot up . . . [that] normalize[s] drug use and facilitate[s] addiction by sending a powerful message to teenagers that the government thinks illegal drugs can be used safely."[25]

A public health perspective on overdose prevention sites starts with the evidence. One important study found a 35% reduction in overdose deaths near the Vancouver supervised consumption facility, greater than reductions in other parts of the city.[26] Sites provide an access point to effective treatment[27] and other social services.[28] There is also evidence of other community benefits from overdose prevention sites. Research has found declines in the number of syringes in neighborhoods near these facilities, and in reports of public drug use.[29]

Scientists disagree about the quality of evidence supporting supervised consumption facilities. However, even when some have found the impact of these sites to be "uncertain," they have not disagreed with "continuing to test and develop" these programs "in locations where public injecting and drug-related harms are a major problem."[30] Moreover, there is no evidence to support the idea that establishing these facilities induces teenagers to use drugs; in a rapid response to the deputy attorney general's words, the Association of Schools and Programs in Public Health stated:

> The experience of other countries show that safe injection sites do not increase drug use in the area—in fact, crime and public nuisance decrease in the areas around these programs. . . . Research shows that people who use supervised sites take better care of themselves, reduce or eliminate their needle sharing, use their drugs more safely, and ultimately reduce their drug use.[31]

A number of US cities are now considering opening overdose prevention sites.[32]

What is the medical use of heroin?

The medical use of heroin is an approach for people with the most difficulty stabilizing their opioid addiction in response to usual treatment, including adequate doses of methadone. Several European countries, including England, Switzerland, and the Netherlands, offer heroin as treatment on the grounds that taking this opioid in a controlled environment, often twice or 3 times a day, is preferable to using drugs under dangerous circumstances on the streets.

Medical heroin clinics have strict policies for entry and discharge. To qualify, individuals must have failed other treatments, including methadone. Patients may be asked to agree to specific rules of the clinic, including showing up on time, cleaning up after using heroin, and not creating a nuisance in the community upon leaving.

At Swiss clinics for medical heroin, physicians prescribe a dose of opioids (measured in milligrams of morphine) for each patient. Each day, the patient can ask for some or all of the dose to be taken as (1) pharmaceutical-grade heroin; or (2) as methadone, or (3) as a combination of them both. The clinics prepare the doses, but the patients inject themselves. Patients leave soon afterwards, walking out of nondescript office buildings located on blocks with restaurants, florists, and other community businesses. At clinics in England, individuals are permitted to take heroin home to use.

Evidence from multiple studies suggests that stable doses of medical heroin can help individuals stay in treatment, use fewer illicit drugs, commit fewer crimes, and achieve greater housing stability. Moreover, in Swiss trials, nearly two-thirds of patients had transitioned to methadone treatment alone within 5 years.[33] There is limited interest at the moment in establishing this type of harm reduction approach in the United States.

What limits the expansion of harm reduction programs in the United States?

Despite ample evidence that harm reduction programs save lives, their rate of adoption remains quite low in the United States. For every police department embracing the use of naloxone, there are several others that have not seen fit to do so. A study published by the Centers for Disease Control and Prevention in August 2018 found that bystanders were present in 44% of fatal overdoses but seldom used naloxone.[34]

Many communities fight the establishment of treatment programs, syringe services programs, and other harm reduction services on the grounds that they would lower property values or only make matters worse, despite ample evidence to the contrary. As of mid-2018, there are no officially sanctioned overdose prevention sites in the United States.

What explains so many missed opportunities to save lives? One clue can be found in the definition of harm reduction itself, which includes "a belief in, and respect for, the rights of people who use drugs." To many Americans, drug use and addiction are indicative of a moral failure, not an illness with consequences that can be minimized. Within this mindset, harm reduction programs, by acknowledging the reality of drug use, enables moral failure. Indeed, one recent study found that those who hold stigmatizing attitudes on drug use have particularly low levels of support for harm reduction programs.[35]

Better understanding the nature of addiction as a chronic illness may help change minds about what can be done to save lives. So too would a more broadly accepted sense that treatment and recovery really can return individuals to their families and communities. To those who criticize harm reduction as "enabling," Daniel Raymond of the Harm Reduction Coalition has responded:

True confession: I got into harm reduction to enable people who use drugs. I enable them to protect themselves and their communities from HIV and hepatitis C and overdose. I enable them to feel like they have someone to talk to, someone who cares, someone who respects them and their humanity. I enable them to ask for help and to help others in turn. I enable them to find drug treatment and health care, to reconnect with their families to rebuild their lives. And I enable people who use drugs to take personal responsibility for their health and their futures. If that makes me an enabler, I'm proud to claim that term."[36]

15

CRIMINAL JUSTICE POLICY AND THE OPIOID EPIDEMIC

What is the war on drugs?

The "war on drugs" refers to the primary US approach to addressing drug use since the early 1970s. While its roots can be traced to the anti-drug rhetoric and legislation of the early 20th century, its modern incarnation began with Richard Nixon's campaign for President in 1968. Nixon rallied what he called the "silent majority" against the social transformation of the 1960s. "Just like the plagues and epidemics of former years," he said that drugs "are decimating a generation of Americans."[1]

Once elected, Nixon recognized the problem went beyond the counterculture, affecting thousands of returning Vietnam War veterans. A physician named Jerome Jaffe convinced the president and his advisers that broadly expanding access to addiction treatment was as critical as increasing law enforcement efforts. On June 17, 1971, President Nixon delivered a special message to Congress calling addiction "public enemy number one in the United States" that required "an all-out offensive." He asked Congress for $155 million in new federal funds for the effort.

The first iteration of the war on drugs included a major treatment component. In fact, of the first $155 million, about two-thirds funded treatment. Dr. Jaffe set up an office in the

White House to lead the national response. Working with a staff of more than 100 people, he created the first treatment programs around the country offering a newly appreciated medication, methadone, for individuals with opioid addiction.

The results were unequivocally positive. On September 5, 1972, *The New York Times* cited a substantial decline in New York City's overdose rate, crime rate, and rate of arrestees with drugs in their system in an editorial entitled "Turnaround on Drugs?"[2] In 1972, the FBI reported a 3% reduction in crime nationally, the first decline in nearly two decades. There were major declines in opioid-related deaths in New York, Chicago, Washington, DC, and San Francisco; in the number of emergency department visits due to drugs; and in the number of new hepatitis cases.[3]

This first phase of the war on drugs was short-lived, however. On January 3, 1973, the Governor of New York, Nelson Rockefeller, gave his annual State of the State address. Rockefeller was a generally liberal Republican, but he had national aspirations. He had decided that his path to the top was to get tough on drugs. "The crime, the muggings, the robberies, the murders associated with addiction continue to spread a reign of terror," he declared. "Whole neighborhoods have been as effectively destroyed by addicts as by an invading army. We face the risk of undermining our will as a people—and the ultimate destruction of our society as a whole. This has to stop. This. Is. Going. To. Stop."[4]

Rockefeller proposed a mandatory life sentence without the chance of parole for anyone convicted of selling heroin, methadone, LSD, amphetamines, or marijuana. The New York governor's ideas bolstered those inside the White House who saw the treatment approach as too weak. While Rockefeller's original proposal did not pass, President Nixon adopted the concept of mandatory minimum sentences. When the president began to call for harsh penalties for individuals caught selling drugs, Dr. Jaffe tried to stop him. He wrote in a memo to the president's chief of staff: "While such a bill's appearance of toughness may generate an emotionally based favorable response initially, that reaction is not likely to persist in the face of analyses which show the bill to be counterproductive even in strictly law enforcement terms."[5]

But the die had been cast. The president's aggressive plan went to Congress, and a few weeks later, Dr. Jaffe resigned. From that moment forward, the war on drugs would be known as an enforcement initiative. It would be largely fought—as other wars—with guns.

Federal efforts on drug enforcement expanded even further under President Reagan, whose lead drug adviser was Dr. Carlton Turner, a marijuana researcher at the University of Mississippi. Dr. Turner had made his reputation testifying against marijuana decriminalization laws. He pulled back on support for drug treatment and added more funds to efforts to interrupt the drug trade.[6]

The rise of crack cocaine gave President Reagan and congressional leaders the opportunity to intensify these efforts. In 1986, Congress passed a $1.7 billion bill called the Anti-Drug Abuse Act. The legislation included hundreds of millions of dollars for expensive military equipment to reduce the inflow of drugs, as well as a raft of mandatory minimum sentences for drug possession (including the limit of just 5 grams for crack, compared to 500 grams for cocaine).[7] The bill also included nearly $100 million for new prison construction.

The new law led to "historically unprecedented rates of imprisonment for drug use and possession," according to a committee of the National Research Council, which found that "from 1980 to 2010, the state incarceration rate for drug offenses grew from 15 per 100,000 to more than 140 per 100,000, a faster rate of increase than for any other offense category."[8]

In the Clinton administration, the war on drugs expanded further. The 1994 crime bill created new capital crimes and mandatory sentences and provided for major expansions of state and local police forces. By 1996, more than 1.5 million Americans were arrested for crimes related to drugs. By 1999, two-thirds of the $18 billion spent by the federal government on drug control went to enforcement and interdiction.[9] This pattern would continue for two more decades.

Has the war on drugs failed?

Yes. In recent years, one of the nation's most respected scientific organizations, the National Research Council of the National Academy of Sciences, Engineering and Medicine, reviewed hundreds of studies on the enforcement of drug laws. These studies covered both military and police efforts to reduce the supply of drugs and enforcement efforts to arrest people who use drugs. Pointing out that "the ultimate objective of both supply and demand side enforcement efforts is to reduce the consumption of illicit drugs," a 2014 report found that "there is little evidence that enforcement efforts have been successful in this regard."

While noting limitations of the data, the report also concluded that "the best empirical evidence suggests that the successive iterations of the war on drugs—through a substantial public policy effort—are unlikely to have markedly or clearly reduced drug crime over the past three decades."

Many scientific studies have explored what went wrong. These studies illustrate the resilience of the drug market, which tends to keep prices affordable even as interdiction efforts, drug seizures, and other police activities rise. For example, the median price of heroin per gram fell by 93% between 1981 and 2007 despite enormous enforcement efforts.[10] "If production is stopped in Country A, then it might automatically soar in Country B," explained one expert.[11]

A 2018 report from the Pew Charitable Trusts noted the jump in the number of Americans in prison from drug offenses from fewer than 25,000 in 1980 to more than 300,000 today. Yet the Pew analysis found that the states with more people in prison did not have less drug use, arrests, or overdose deaths. "For instance," the report explained, "Tennessee imprisoned drug offenders at more than three times the rate of New Jersey, but the states' rates of self-reported drug use are virtually the same."[12]

Even where an intensive law enforcement crackdown might appear to be successful, research has found that "displacement of the drug and crime problem was a common problem," with drug use reappearing elsewhere or after the response subsided.[13]

Beyond not achieving its desired goals, the drug war has created new problems. What happens when so many are incarcerated for so long? One major risk is continued drug use. That's in part because many become or remain addicted to substances available behind bars. It's also because individuals in jails and prisons can be recruited to gangs and other criminal organizations, which, in turn, strengthens their ability to distribute drugs. Incarceration also reduces the ability of people to stabilize their lives and break free from drugs, as having a criminal record undermines opportunities for legitimate employment after release.

At a global scale, the drug war has strengthened criminal organizations, contributed to public corruption, and sparked violence—fostering the conditions for social disorder and drug use. "The high black market price for illegal drugs has generated huge profits for the groups that produce and sell them," wrote President Reagan's former Secretary of State George Shultz with the former Mexican Finance Minister Pedro Aspe in The New York Times. They explained that the resulting income "is invested in buying state-of-the-art weapons, hiring gangs to defend their trade, paying off public officials and making drugs easily available to children, to get them addicted."[14]

Indeed, in multiple US cities, including Detroit and Baltimore, the drug trade has led not only to the growth of violent gangs and thousands of resulting homicides but also to police corruption and civil rights violations. In Mexico and Central America, gang violence related to drugs is responsible for more than 100,000 deaths and drives many in fear to migrate to the United States. The drug war in Afghanistan has empowered the Taliban.

At the community level, the drug war backfires every time a person who uses drugs is afraid to seek assistance at a syringe services or a treatment program. The lost opportunity for engagement means a greater likelihood of continued drug use, as well as a larger risk of passing HIV and other infectious diseases to others. A comprehensive review published in the *Lancet* found that strict enforcement of harsh drug laws is linked to syringe sharing and HIV infection.[15]

At a cost of more than $1 trillion, the enforcement efforts of the drug war have pulled resources from our nation's other priorities, including improving education, ameliorating poverty, providing healthcare to those in need—and for that matter, even lowering taxes to boost the economy. To the extent that such efforts would have created hope and reduced despair for millions of Americans, the result has been greater drug use than otherwise would have occurred.

It is no wonder that historian Michael Massing concluded, "It would be hard to think of an area of U.S. social policy that has failed more completely than the war on drugs."[16]

What is the role of race in the war on drugs?

In 2014, the National Research Council documented the enormous growth of incarceration in the United States, which it found to be "historically unprecedented and internationally unique." About 1 in 4 of the world's prisoners are held in the United States, where just 1 in 20 people in the world live. The US rate of incarceration is 5 to 10 times higher than in comparable Western European nations.[17]

The burden of excess incarceration has not been equally distributed. The National Research Council found, "More than half the prison population is black or Hispanic. . . . In

2010, blacks were incarcerated at six times and Hispanics at three times the rate for non-Hispanic whites."[18] As Michelle Alexander has written in *The New Jim Crow*, "The racial dimension of mass incarceration is its most striking feature. No other country in the world imprisons so many of its racial and ethnic minorities."[19]

The major reason for the high rates of incarceration in general—and for the extraordinarily high rates of incarceration of minorities—are patterns in arrest and incarceration rates for drugs, which have been between 3 and 6 times higher for African Americans than for whites. Alexander has noted that "convictions for drug offenses are the single most important cause of the explosion in incarceration rates in the United States."[20]

What accounts for this major difference? Not drug use, which is about the same for African Americans and whites. "There is also little evidence, when all drug types are considered, that blacks sell drugs more often than whites," the National Research Council report found.[21] Rather, those types of drugs most often used and sold by minority communities face the most aggressive enforcement and the stiffest criminal penalties.

Inequity in incarceration has had a devastating impact on millions of individuals and their families and on thousands of neighborhoods. Millions of people have been arrested, charged, and given little opportunity to mount a defense, with convictions carrying a host of legal consequences—including prohibitions on voting, living in public housing, and qualifying for certain jobs.

The result has been a profound disenfranchisement of minority communities. "An extraordinary percentage of black men in the United States are legally barred from voting today, just as they have been throughout most of American history," Alexander wrote. "They are also subject to legalized discrimination in employment, housing, education, public benefits, and jury services, just as their parents, grandparents, and great-grandparents once were."[22]

The vast disparities central to the enforcement of drug laws has led the National Academies of Sciences, Engineering and Medicine to conclude that "the disparate impact of the war on drugs on communities of color and high rates of incarceration for drug offenses among African Americans and Hispanics make a reduction in drug-related incarceration an urgent priority."[23]

Is the war on drugs over?

No. The nation's response to the opioid epidemic reflects a conflicted mix of treatment efforts and a resurgence in certain types of enforcement efforts. In many jurisdictions, for example, police and prosecutors are turning overdoses into crime scenes, looking to charge those involved in drug activity with homicide. The targets are not just drug kingpins. As *The New York Times* reported, "Using laws devised to go after drug dealers, [prosecutors] are charging friends, partners and siblings. The accused include young people who shared drugs at a party and a son who gave his mother heroin after her pain medication had been cut off. Many are fellow users, themselves struggling with addiction."[24]

Some good news is passage in late 2018 of criminal justice reform, which rolled back a number of severe penalties related to drugs that have been in place since the mid-1990s. Such progress, however, is likely to be fragile. The overdose crisis has led to state and federal proposals to increase drug penalties, including mandatory minimum sentencing, for possession and distribution of fentanyl. And aggressive rhetoric still permeates discussion of drug policy. In 2017, the president of the United States told President Rodrigo Duterte of the Philippines he was doing "an unbelievable job on the drug problem."[25] Duterte has led a campaign of brutal killings of thousands of people with addiction.[26]

How can police departments address the opioid epidemic?

In April 2018, a small number of public health experts and municipal police chiefs came together at the offices of the Police Executive Research Forum in Washington, DC, to develop a list of 10 "standards of care" for police departments on opioids.[27] The group included two former leaders of the White House Office of National Drug Control Policy, several faculty from Johns Hopkins University, and police chiefs from Burlington, Vermont; Arlington, Massachusetts; and Morgantown, West Virginia.

The first recommended standard of care was to "focus on overdose deaths." That is, police departments should keep their eyes on the prize of saving lives—and not be diverted by placing undue importance on less important measures, such as the number of arrests. A promising model exists in New York City, where the police and health departments have adapted the successful CompStat model to reduce overdose into a process known as RxStat.[28]

The second standard of care is to provide the overdose reversal medication naloxone to every police officer, along with training on how to reverse an overdose. Studies have found that police officers have used naloxone to save thousands of lives, with training and experience increasing their comfort and confidence. However, only several hundred police departments (of the thousands in the country) routinely provide this medication for their officers to carry.

The third standard of care is to educate officers and the public about addiction and stigma, using personal narratives of recovery as well as data about the effectiveness of treatment.

The fourth standard is to refer to treatment as an alternative to arrest. There are several promising models in which police departments find people in need of assistance and send them for help instead of to jail. One example is the Law Enforcement Assisted Diversion (LEAD) program, first launched in Seattle in 2011. Police officers trained in this approach refer individuals to case managers who provide access to treatment and other services. An initial analysis found that participants had "60% lower odds of arrest at six months post program entry and 58% and 29% lower odds of arrest and being charged with a felony, respectively at three years post program entry."[29]

LEAD is one of several promising programs. In Arlington, Massachusetts, police officers work directly with clinicians to reach affected individuals. In Gloucester, Massachusetts, the police department is a safe place for users interested in accessing treatment to go. Manchester, New Hampshire, and Annapolis, Maryland, are other cities that have adopted a similar "safe stations" model for their fire departments.

The fifth and sixth standards for police departments called for law enforcement leaders to advocate for broad expansions to effective treatment inside and outside of the correctional system. "Without such access," the group wrote, "diversion programs will have limited success, and recidivism will remain high.

The seventh standard strongly endorsed well-managed syringe services programs as critical to reducing HIV, hepatitis C, and other infectious diseases, as well as reducing the risk of needle-stick injuries for police officers. The eighth and ninth standards encouraged police departments to discuss fentanyl checking programs and overdose prevention sites with their local communities. Finally, the tenth standard of care called for police departments to support strong legal protections (known as good samaritan laws) for individuals who call 911 in the setting of an overdose.

What about enforcement efforts? A systematic review found that reactive "crackdowns" were not effective, but that "proactive and partnership policing" focused on drug trafficking and crime prevention through changes to the physical structure of communities (such as eliminating vacant housing) had the best records of success.[30]

Putting it all together, the Pew Charitable Trusts found:

The most effective response to drug misuse is a combination of law enforcement to curtail trafficking and prevent the emergence of new markets, alternative sentencing to divert nonviolent drug offenders from costly imprisonment; treatment to reduce dependency and recidivism, and prevention efforts that can identify individuals at high risk for substance use disorders.[31]

How can jails and prisons address the opioid epidemic?

Every day in the United States, thousands of people with opioid addiction are arrested on a wide range of charges. Only a small minority will receive treatment of any kind in detention. Of those who receive treatment, fewer than 5% will receive the effective medications methadone or buprenorphine.[32]

The nation's correctional system is not just a missed opportunity to treat opioid addiction; it is contributing to death from overdose. That's not only because some people die in jails and prisons as a result of the dehydration associated with withdrawal.[33] It's also because people with opioid addiction lose their tolerance to opioids while incarcerated. Upon release, if they return to their previous dose of prescription opioids or heroin, they are at risk for a fatal overdose. The risk of fatal overdose is more than 100 times greater for someone who has been recently released from detention than for the general population.[34]

The risk of fatal overdose after release from detention is dramatically reduced with effective treatment. After the State of Rhode Island offered everyone in the state's jail and prison access to all three Food and Drug Administration–approved medications and connected them to treatment in the community upon release, the number of overdose deaths among people released dropped by 60%.[35] Treatment also reduces the chance of criminal recidivism.[36] However, even though the President's Advisory Commission recommended access to treatment with medications for everyone in pretrial detention,[37] and even though the American Correctional Association has endorsed broad access to treatment in the justice system,[38] this care remains very much the exception rather than the rule in the United States.

Why don't more jails and prisons offer access to opioid addiction treatment?

In addition to inadequate understanding of addiction and insufficient resources, many wardens are highly skeptical of providing effective addiction treatment. That's because their primary experience with opioid addiction may be the illicit market for drugs within their own facilities. Their primary effort to shut down this market may be to try to catch people smuggling contraband. In many places, this battle has focused on buprenorphine, one form of which is a thin film that can be easily hidden.

The street market for buprenorphine is unique. Most people who have tried buprenorphine without a prescription report that they take it to reduce heroin use or avoid going into withdrawal.[39] Taking diverted buprenorphine is associated with having attempted, and failed, to obtain treatment with this medication.[40] For this reason, some prosecutors, such as those in Burlington, Vermont, have decided not to press charges against people found to have non-prescribed buprenorphine in their possession.[41]

Yet in the context of smuggling, jail and prison officials generally see buprenorphine as no different from heroin or oxycodone. In fact, the smuggling of buprenorphine has driven some correctional officials to distraction. They swap stories of how the contraband has entered their facilities ("In a Bible, doctor, I swear"). They purchase expensive surveillance technology and conduct elaborate sting operations. Some have gone so far as to try to ban visitors from giving inmates books to read.[42]

Correctional officials rarely recognize that the illicit market for buprenorphine in detention exists because of limited access to treatment. (Some public health officials have tried to explain to them that if jails and prisons did not serve meals, people would smuggle in food.) Jails and prisons can substantially reduce or eliminate the demand for contraband buprenorphine by treating opioid addiction effectively. Doing so would save many lives in the process.

Fortunately, some correctional facilities are breaking free from past practice, expanding access to treatment, and seeing positive results.[43] More change may be coming. Failing to treat the disease of addiction is a likely violation of both the 8th Amendment to the Constitution's prohibition on cruel and unusual punishment as well as the rights of inmates under the Americans with Disabilities Act.[44] In November 2018, a federal judge in Massachusetts ordered the Essex County Jail to continue treating an inmate with methadone, rather than follow the usual policy of weaning him off of the medication.[45]

What are drug courts?

Drug courts are specialized courts that are referred nonviolent cases. There are as many types of drug courts are there are state and local judicial systems.

When working well, a drug court program can offer participants effective treatment as an alternative to incarceration. However, this is more the exception than the rule. Some drug courts place people in treatment programs that do not offer treatment with effective medications; others limit medication options to naltrexone, which is far from the most appropriate choice for all patients. Very few participants in drug courts are referred to programs that offer all three Food and Drug Administration–approved medications: naltrexone, methadone, and buprenorphine. In fact, some judges and drug court programs have ordered people to stop taking methadone or buprenorphine, increasing their chance for relapse and overdose.

Some drug courts become quite punitive when patients relapse, even if just one time, requiring them to serve long prison sentences. In extreme cases, the sentences can turn out longer than if the individual had not been sent to drug court in the first place. A better approach is to recognize that the best response to relapse is continued treatment; many patients in effective treatment programs go on to achieve a sustained remission.

Drug courts are just one piece of the solution to the opioid epidemic. For many people, diversion to treatment before arrest or conviction is likely to make more sense than drug court. Individuals whose only apparent violation is drug possession can be referred to effective treatment without their ever being arrested, going to jail, and acquiring a criminal record.

What can the United States learn from other countries' approaches to criminal justice policy?

In the late 1990s, Portugal faced a crisis related to addiction. After the long dictatorship of Antonio de Oliviera Salazar ended, drug use exploded, and the country struggled to contain the consequences. Rather than committing to a strategy based on enforcement, however, Portugal took an entirely different approach.

In 2001, Portugal decriminalized possession of small amounts of drugs—all drugs—while continuing to enforce laws against trafficking. Portugal then endorsed a wide range of harm reduction activities. These included syringe services programs to reduce the spread of infectious disease, overdose prevention sites to prevent overdose deaths, and—most of all—treatment programs that utilized effective medications. Individuals who misuse drugs can be brought for assessment and triage and offered services.[46] Those not interested in treatment can still receive methadone on a daily basis via a mobile service that engages users and provides multiple opportunities for them to seek more organized care.

A decade later, the results are in. Portugal has seen declining rates of drug use (particularly among adolescents), increases in the number of people seeking treatment, and reductions in HIV infections. Overdose deaths fell 75% to a grand total of 12 deaths for the nation in 2012.[47]

How was Portugal able to pivot to a public health approach to addiction? "Every family had its own drug addict. It was so, so present in everyday life, that it turned public opinion," the nation's top official for the drug problem told *National Public Radio*. "We are dealing with a chronic relapsing disease, and this is a disease like any other. I do not put a diabetic in jail, for instance."[48]

Other European countries have also embraced harm reduction and addiction treatment as alternatives to a law enforcement response to addiction. France saw an 80% drop in overdose deaths as it scaled up treatment with buprenorphine.[49] Barcelona, Spain, has nearly 3 times the population of Baltimore, Maryland, but just 10% of the overdose deaths. One key has been a network of overdose prevention sites that offer intensive counseling, methadone, infectious disease care, and other services.

To be fair, Europe has yet to see the influx of fentanyl and its analogues recently seen in the United States. But by addressing opioid addiction as a health crisis, these countries are far better prepared for whatever drug challenge comes next.

16

SURVEILLANCE, EVALUATION, AND RESEARCH AND THE OPIOID EPIDEMIC

How well is the United States tracking the opioid epidemic?

Not well. For a threat that has cost tens of thousands of lives and reduced US life expectancy, the opioid crisis is not sufficiently monitored. Federal reports with data on the number of fatal overdoses are released 6 months to a year after deaths actually occur. Many states and localities rely on a patchwork of coroners and medical examiners, who may apply different criteria to decide whether to call a death an overdose.[1] Death certificates in cases of overdose may miss as many as half of deaths associated with heroin.[2]

Data beyond the number of fatal overdoses are also difficult to come by. While some cities can find out from their emergency medical systems how many nonfatal overdoses occurred in the previous week, others do not learn how many occurred until months later, if ever. Few places track the number of people receiving any treatment for addiction, let alone the number of people receiving evidence-based care. Some prescription drug monitoring programs produce reports on opioid prescribing, but these can be so broad in scope it may be unclear to understand whether prescribing is getting better or worse. There is little sharing of data by law enforcement agencies about the changing nature of the drug supply; this has limited the recognition of rapid shifts towards fentanyl in some markets.

There are a few reasons why useful data on the opioid epidemic is so scarce. The US system for tracking the cause of all deaths is notoriously weak, relying on death certificates filled out by thousands of different people using varying standards. As far as non-fatal overdoses, in the early 2000s, the federal government decided to cut back on funding a major surveillance system that tracked emergency room visits related to use of illicit drugs.[3] (This proved to be terrible timing.)

Meanwhile, data on treatment are held by thousands of different programs and payers without a central tracking mechanism, with significant limitations on data sharing under federal law. Many specialty addiction treatment programs also still operate with paper and pencil patient records, so are unable to quickly share electronic health information even if they were permitted to do so. The federal funding that Congress provided several years ago to advance electronic medical records did not include support addiction treatment providers.

A major consequence of poor data is ill-informed policy. Without a real sense of whether the crisis is getting better or worse in their areas in their areas, many states and localities may find it easy to stick with traditional strategies for treatment and law enforcement that are unsupported by evidence. Without the ability to see results, it is unlikely that politicians will invest in promising initiatives that do not have a vocal political constituency, such as law enforcement diversion programs and treatment programs in jails and prisons.

That's why information on the opioid crisis is more than numbers on a page. It is essential to progress.

What trends related to the opioid epidemic are most useful to monitor?

One of the first states to establish an effective public "dashboard" on opioids—a central repository of critical data related to the epidemic—was Rhode Island. A team of researchers at Brown University started this process in 2015 by releasing some hard facts about the epidemic in the state. These facts included that there were more overdose deaths in Rhode Island than homicides, suicides, and motor vehicle fatalities—combined.[4]

The expert team then issued a call for written comments and held several public meetings to gather ideas about what the state might do to respond to the opioid epidemic. The result was a plan with specific metrics for success. To track these metrics, and with support from the Centers for Disease Control and Prevention, Rhode Island produced a public dashboard.

At http://preventoverdoseRI.org, the state displays the number of overdoses by month. Data are also available for individual cities and towns. The dashboard describes the types of drugs that contribute to the problem, exposing a shift over the last several years from prescription opioids to heroin and then fentanyl. It also tracks the number of overdose victims who died after release from jail or prison. (This measure is linked to successful state efforts to provide treatment in detention).

Rhode Island tracks the number of emergency department visits for overdose, and the state maps where these overdoses occurred. The state measures access to the reversal drug naloxone, both in the hospital and the community. There are also data on the number of people receiving effective treatment, including treatment with methadone and buprenorphine. To improve physician prescribing, Rhode Island tracks the number of people receiving opioids for the first time, and the number who receive both opioids and benzodiazepines such as alprazolam (Xanax®)—a potentially deadly combination.

It is no surprise that Rhode Island's governor is Gina Raimondo, a former management consultant. The dashboard's value stems not just from its clarity and public accessibility but also from its close connection to the state's plan. Several states and localities are following similar approaches, using public comment and expert input to identify evidence-based strategies—and then establishing tracking mechanisms to assure that they are working.

What other trends make sense to track?

Current approaches to tracking the opioid epidemic are limited by what data are available. Looking ahead, it is possible to imagine the collection of additional information to guide local, state, and national responses to the crisis. New measures might assess:

- *The stigma of addiction.* Many people hold intensely negative feelings about addiction; these attitudes complicate efforts to pursue effective policy. Researchers are developing approaches to measuring stigma.[5] Doing so on a regular basis would encourage greater efforts to address this problem.
- *Effective transitions in care.* Many people begin addiction treatment in one setting and then move to another. For example, those who receive their first dose of buprenorphine in the emergency department must transition to an available provider for ongoing care; those who begin in a residential treatment program must find ongoing services in the community. Measuring access to care across different settings would bring attention to the need for greater coordination and to gaps in the system of care.
- *Innovations in law enforcement.* Some city and county police departments are making important strides against the opioid epidemic—and others are pursuing enforcement approaches that are making the epidemic worse. How are local residents to know the difference? A measure of what's happening with arrests and diversion to effective treatment would help.
- *Success in prevention.* A set of measures for youth opportunity and resilience would help communities recognize the importance of a broad set of investments to prevent addiction.
- *Support for recovery.* The success of people in stopping opioid misuse often depends on their finding jobs,

locating safe and affordable housing, and accessing peer support. Measures that assess how well a community assists people in recovery to put their lives back together would spur greater investment in such approaches.

What is the role of evaluation in assessing the response to the opioid epidemic?

Evaluation assesses whether a specific response to the opioid crisis is effective. Evaluation can be distinguished from monitoring, which refers to tracking changes in key measures of the epidemic over time. Communities should seek ways to support evaluation of key efforts to be sure what they are doing is working.

Many communities assess their own programs by comparing what happened before with what happened after implementation. This form of evaluation, often called "pre–post," is relatively weak, because coincidental factors might actually be responsible for the change. A stronger methodology is to use a comparison group.

For example, some have claimed that naloxone increases overdose deaths, based on the fact that states that recently passed naloxone laws experience more overdoses than states that do not.[6] The problem with this "pre–post" reasoning, however, is that states pass naloxone laws *because* they have a problem with rising overdose deaths.

A better designed evaluation compared the changes in overdose in those Massachusetts communities that expanded access to naloxone with the changes in overdose in similar Massachusetts communities that did not. This study found a substantial reduction in deaths associated with the naloxone distribution program.[7]

The best type of comparison involves a random assignment, so that the only difference between people who received an intervention and those who did not is pure chance. For many policies and programs, however, this type of research design is not possible. For example, it may be illegal (and unethical) to expand benefits for important health services to some people but not others.

In other cases, random assignment might well be possible. For example, if a program to help people in recovery find employment were to have more applicants than spots, officials might use a lottery to pick the participants. An evaluation could compare the job outcomes of those who were selected with those who were not.

Because of limitations in time, effort, and resources, it is not feasible to conduct evaluations on every part of the response to the opioid epidemic. Communities should therefore think about where having solid information will be most useful. For example, a city may have a new idea for an outreach team to connect with people at high risk of overdose and may be able to convince a local philanthropy to fund a pilot effort. An evaluation by a local university researcher could inform a decision later about whether to continue or end the pilot program. It might also provide information useful to other communities struggling to reach a similar population.

What are some of the most promising areas of current research related to opioids and opioid addiction?

In July 2018, writing in the *Journal of the American Medical Association*, the director of the National Institutes of Health, Dr. Francis Collins, and the director of the National Institutes on Drug Abuse, Dr. Nora Volkow, set out a $500 million plan for research on the opioid epidemic. The plan focuses on improving treatments for pain and improving treatments for opioid addiction.[8]

With respect to pain, the National Institutes of Health hopes to find ways to stop short-term discomfort from developing into chronic pain. Another goal: finding therapies that address pain without stimulating the reward and pleasure systems. In theory, at least, such therapies should pose much less of a risk for addiction than currently available opioids.

For opioid addiction, the National Institutes of Health's goal is to identify new and more effective types of treatments, as well as new types of reversal medications that potentially can last longer in the body than naloxone. The effort also seeks to find ways to better use existing therapies. The agency is planning to study innovative models of care in hospitals, jails, and other community locations—models that provide medications along with other key services to support treatment success and recovery.

Outside of this federal effort, there is a major focus on studying the treatment and care of babies born with neonatal abstinence syndrome, including assessing whether specialized services can avoid developmental delay and school problems. Local agencies and foundations are looking into new harm reduction approaches. Researchers are beginning to assess the value of "checking" programs that allow people who use illicit drugs to know what they are taking. There is early evidence that these programs may help reduce the risks of death from fentanyl.[9] Other areas of investigation include the use of overdose prevention sites and the addition of new services, including initiation of addiction treatment, to syringe services programs.

As communities mobilize to do more for prevention and recovery, local, well-designed evaluations will differentiate what works from what does not, potentially giving more confidence to policymakers eager to make non-traditional investments.

A critical area for further research is stigma. That's because the stigma on addiction impedes the adoption of many types of effective policies, reduces access to a variety of needed services, and even keeps people with opioid addiction from seeking help. Some important questions include the origin of stigma, and what works to counter the effects of stigma on policies, programs, families, and individuals.

What are the challenges to moving research discoveries quickly into practice?

In 2015, researchers from Yale University published a randomized controlled trial on the treatment of opioid addiction. The study asked whether patients in the emergency department would benefit from prompt access to buprenorphine, including onsite prior to discharge. The researchers were asking not what, how, why, or who—but where.

The results of their study were that patients who received access to buprenorphine in the emergency department were twice as likely to remain engaged in treatment 30 days later compared with those who just received a referral to treatment. Given the magnitude of the opioid crisis, the Yale study should have caused an earthquake in clinical medicine. Instead, it registered barely a tremor.[10] For years after publication, few emergency departments in the United States routinely offered access to this treatment. Even now, there is only a steady trickle of interest.

What is taking so long? In healthcare, inertia rules. Many doctors practice the way they were trained to do so, unable to keep up rapidly with advances in care. Some experts in the field have estimated that the average time for a research discovery to make it to the bedside is 17 years.[11]

With respect to policy and programs, too, health administrators tend to stick with what is comfortable. Many people are hired to do specific tasks, not to change them as evidence advances. There is often a far greater fear of an error of commission (doing something wrong) than an error of omission (not doing something right).

For example, new evidence is emerging that providing people who use drugs with devices to check for fentanyl can reduce their risks of a fatal overdose. Some people will look at these data, see the fentanyl epidemic that is claiming more than 20,000 lives a year, and argue that there is an urgent need to pilot and evaluate this technology. Others, however, will look at the same data, see an unproven technology, worry about unforeseen adverse effects, and think: How about we wait a bit?

This inherent conservatism of policymakers was a major roadblock to the development of new therapies for the AIDS epidemic. Thirty years ago, with few treatments available for this dreaded new infection, patients and their loved ones revolted. On October 11, 1988, thousands of protesters from the organization AIDS Coalition to Unleash Power (ACT UP) descended on the Food and Drug Administration and demanded greater access to promising treatments.[12] Hundreds of people were arrested, and coverage of the protest led newscasts across the country. Similar protests at the National Institutes of Health called for greater inclusion of a diversity of patients in research planning and trial design. Advocacy by ACT UP contributed to major changes at both agencies and a period of rapid innovation in treatment options.

There's no iron law that great ideas, even those that are proven to work, become widely adopted. Pressure informed by evidence from elected officials, families, clinicians, and individuals with opioid addiction themselves may be necessary for the country to fully embrace public health approaches and get better results.

17

WHAT TO DO FOR THE OPIOID EPIDEMIC

What can the addiction field do to address the opioid epidemic?

The addiction field is large and diverse, stretching from small mutual support groups to large treatment programs. This diversity is both a strength and a weakness. A variety of treatment and recovery options and settings for individuals with opioid addiction are very much needed. However, significant variability in quality remains a stubborn problem, with many programs using ineffective and even counterproductive approaches. Another concern is that the majority of specialty addiction programs operate on an outdated model built around brief episodes of care. In the midst of an epidemic, the addiction field must modernize.

Change is needed in mutual support groups, which can offer vital support for people in treatment and recovery. Peers offer a unique level of understanding and assistance distinct from treatment professionals. Unfortunately, many of these groups refuse to include people taking medications for opioid addiction, asserting that such people are not in "true recovery." The result is that some people refuse to take medications, increasing their risk for fatal overdose and relapse.

Residential treatment programs can develop and enforce professional standards that separate high-quality programs from those that cost a fortune and deliver a pittance. There are agencies that accredit these programs; stronger standards and greater transparency would provide far more confidence and credibility for the industry.

Outpatient treatment programs vary widely as well. Some clinics struggle with the labels of "pill mills" or "gas and go," reflecting little in the way of services other than providing medications. One poorly managed clinic that offers methadone can confuse an entire city into thinking that expanding access to an effective medication is a misguided approach. Programs that offer a range of services with excellent quality can advocate strongly both for adequate reimbursement and for high standards of care.

Traditionally, the addiction field has existed as a world unto itself. The opioid epidemic demands that those who are most knowledgeable and experienced about addiction—including those with lived experience—share their stories to dispel stigma and to inform local and national policy. Those in the addiction field have a special opportunity to amplify the voice of people in treatment and recovery.

What can others in the healthcare system do?

Others in the healthcare system—including clinicians without expertise in addiction medicine, insurers, and leaders of healthcare organizations—can start by looking in the mirror. The current opioid epidemic has much of its roots in the massive increase in prescriptions of pain medications—a surge that was followed by an explosion in the use of heroin and fentanyl. With a sense of responsibility, the healthcare system can work to become less of the problem and more of the solution.

Less of the problem

The first step is for doctors to prescribe opioids only when necessary. Insurers can improve coverage of alternative treatments for pain, clinicians can learn when to recommend them, and patients and families can educate themselves about their value.

When opioids are the best choice, physicians can prescribe what is needed and not more. The Food and Drug Administration (FDA), health systems, professional associations, and others can create and promote clear recommendations, based on evidence, on the use of opioids in specific clinical situations, such as after particular types of surgeries. Electronic prescribing systems can default to these settings.

In extreme cases, authorities can step in to stop clinicians who prescribe opioids excessively for pain from placing patients at risk. The FDA can review, warn, and if necessary, revoke authority to prescribe particularly high-risk medications, such as fentanyl. Boards of medicine and nursing can respond promptly to allegations of practice far outside the standard of care.

When patients need opioids for long-term pain, for cancer or otherwise, they should be allowed to take them. Abruptly discontinuing or lowering the dose of opioid medications for otherwise stable patients can trigger withdrawal, significant pain, and despair—even to the point of suicide.

More of the solution

Atonement means more than an apology; it requires making things right. The healthcare system can take advantage of an enormous opportunity crystallized by the following statistic from the US Surgeon General: Only about 1 in 10 Americans with addiction receives treatment.

Insurers can cover FDA-approved therapies for opioid addiction without arbitrary limits or roadblocks. (To afford this policy, they can stop paying for residential treatment programs that do not follow evidence or best practices). Clinicians in all settings can learn to diagnose addiction, start therapy (if appropriate), and refer (if necessary) for ongoing care or for treatment by specialists. Primary care clinics can develop comprehensive programs to treat patients with addiction, just as they have efforts for diabetes or heart failure. And specialty addiction treatment programs can be incentivized and supported to incorporate primary care services into their treatment settings for particularly complex patients, similarly to how specialty heart failure clinics or HIV clinics have become the primary care providers for high-need patients with complex and challenging conditions.

Hospitals and health systems can offer addiction treatment services in emergency departments, on the wards, and in their outpatient centers. If there are not enough high-quality specialty addiction programs in their communities, health systems can do what they would do for any other condition taking so many lives: open new programs themselves.

Professional education can play a central role in transforming US healthcare. Medical and nursing students can learn about the biology of addiction, how it is treated, and their future role in mitigating the effects of the opioid epidemic. Postgraduate training programs—such as residencies in internal medicine, family medicine, and psychiatry—can assure that their graduates have experience with appropriate pain management and effective addiction treatment and are ready to be part of the solution from the moment they start practicing on their own.

What can the criminal justice system do?

The opioid epidemic involves a series of vicious cycles within the criminal justice system. These include:

- When people with opioid addiction are arrested for non-violent offenses such as drug possession, they may lose their jobs, their housing, and their health coverage. This makes it far less likely they will succeed in treatment and be able to achieve and sustain remission and recovery.

- When jails and prisons require people with opioid addiction to go through withdrawal and lose their tolerance to opioids, there is a far greater risk of fatal overdose when use starts again.
- When judges order inmates into "treatment" that does not offer effective medications, the chance of failure is high. As a result, drug courts can wind up reinforcing the stigma on treatment and on addiction at the same time.

Breaking these vicious cycles requires major changes in policing, prosecution, adjudication, parole, and probation.

Police departments can follow the "standards of care" put together by law enforcement and public health experts.[1] These include carrying naloxone, diverting more people from arrest to treatment, supporting syringe exchange programs, and recognizing the value in harm reduction approaches. There is also a leadership opportunity for police departments to help their communities rethink their approach to the epidemic. In Burlington, Vermont, for example, the local police chief has said that just arresting everyone for drug use is counterproductive. He has called for expanding access to easily accessible treatment across the correctional system and in syringe services programs.[2]

Prosecutors can take as their goals not the number of arrests and prosecutions, but rather the community harms of overdose, property crime, and homelessness. Judges can educate themselves about the evidence on treatment medications and insist that programs affiliated with their courts offer a full spectrum of treatment options. Parole and probation systems can develop referral relationships with the highest-quality treatment providers in their jurisdictions and organize a variety of services to support individuals in recovery.

The criminal justice system can also resist the temptation to backslide. How easy it is to announce a "zero tolerance" policy, to lead a raid that arrests dozens of people who use drugs, to criticize a syringe services program for "sending the wrong message," or to demand that people who use opioids change their behavior immediately. But such steps will only make it more difficult for those with addiction to actually take control of their own lives.

What can litigation do?

A large number of lawsuits from individuals, local governments, and states are seeking to hold major companies in the pharmaceutical industry responsible for the opioid epidemic. If successful, these lawsuits can lead to agreements by companies to stop certain types of marketing, including marketing that would otherwise be allowed under federal law. The lawsuits may also generate substantial sums of funding to address the harms of the epidemic. This funding can support essential, evidence-based efforts to support prevention, treatment, and recovery.

Recently, there has also been litigation against jails and prisons that do not offer effective treatment with medications under the Americans with Disabilities act and the Eighth Amendment. Success can serve to make life-saving care more widely available (and reduce criminal recidivism in the process).

What can local communities do?

Many local communities are on the front lines of the opioid epidemic, with a broad range of tragic consequences in full view: fatal overdoses, theft and violence linked to the illicit drug trade, family disruption, and economic disinvestment.

Other neighborhoods are off the front lines, where it may be possible for many to imagine that the opioid epidemic is not a major threat. It is more likely that these places have the means to hide problems from view, with suffering still happening behind drawn curtains and in the back of ambulances.

There is often resistance in communities of all types to a large-scale response of outreach and treatment. In heavily impacted areas, some may ask: Why does our neighborhood always seem to get the service programs? Why yet another treatment program on our block? In quietly affected areas, some may object to expanding services on the mistaken grounds that "there really isn't a problem here." The result is the same: little action, even when and where it is desperately needed.

One way to avoid this trap is for those affected by the opioid epidemic to talk to their friends and neighbors and, together with first responders and local experts, raise awareness about the opioid crisis and what can be done *here*. And there's a lot that can be done. Neighborhoods can host support groups to bring suffering out of the shadows, establish close relationships with treatment programs, provide education, and make resources available to local residents—such as naloxone kits and cards with information to help people access treatment—that can save lives.

What can cities and counties do?

The rising toll of the opioid epidemic is stressing cities and counties in numerous ways—from the police department to the emergency department, from the school environment to the business climate. Mayors and county executives focused on making progress can ask these seven questions.

Do I have reliable data on the scale of the opioid crisis?

Local elected leaders can work with their police department and local health departments to develop dashboards on emergency department visits, overdose deaths, and services provided. These data can help focus attention on worrisome trends and significant gaps in the system as well as identify when strategies are starting to have an impact.

Are my local clinicians following national standards in prescribing for pain?

Mayors and county executives can obtain commitments from healthcare institutions and large physician practices to adopt key standards, such as the Centers for Disease Control guidelines for the use of opioids for chronic pain. They can also ask healthcare leaders to report on quality metrics that assess whether these guidelines are being followed. These steps can reduce the risk of addiction from excessive prescribing of opioids.

Is there rapid access to evidence-based treatment for opioid addiction?

Treatment that includes medications such as methadone and buprenorphine is associated with a two-thirds or greater reduction in the risk of overdose, greater employment, less infectious disease, and less crime. Yet many healthcare systems do not provide this therapy, and many addiction treatment programs may be following a "detox" or "abstinence only" approach that may actually increase the risk of overdose death upon relapse. Mayors and county executives can convene local hospitals and physician networks, as well as local addiction treatment programs, and ask them to make sure that people in need can access effective services quickly.

Some local governments have taken matters into their own hands. For example, the City of Manchester, New Hampshire, decided to open its firehouses 24/7 to individuals seeking assistance for a drug problem.[3] Hundreds of local residents have shown up to the newly named "safe stations" looking for help. This action has not only provided some direct relief, but it has also given the city a perspective on the gaps in the state's treatment system. Manchester officials are using their experience with "safe stations" to call for a larger investment in effective treatment.

Is my city or county organized to support people in recovery?

Addiction is a chronic illness, and long-term recovery often requires safe housing, employment opportunities, and other supports. Local governments can coordinate services to support individuals in recovery and minimize the chance of relapse.

Can I reduce the burden on law enforcement?

A revolving door of drug arrests for non-violent individuals with opioid addiction is expensive and unhelpful. In fact, many jails force people to withdraw from opioids "cold-turkey," which elevates the risk of fatal overdose upon release. Mayors and county executives can support innovative diversion programs, in which the police and other social service providers connect people to treatment instead of arrest. They can also provide greater access to treatment for those in city and county jails, which can substantially reduce the risk of overdose (and recidivism) upon release.

Can my city or county find ways to engage people who misuse drugs but are not interested in treatment?

For someone with an active opioid addiction, the road to recovery often starts with a baby step. A young man may seek out clean needles in a syringe services program, or a young woman may ask for a way to test drugs for the presence of lethal fentanyl. Each contact is an opportunity to move closer to accepting treatment. Elected leaders can support innovative outreach efforts that reduce the highest-risk behaviors, reduce overdose deaths, and help more people reach treatment and, ultimately, remission and recovery.

Can I reduce the stigma of addiction?

Nobody knows their communities better than locally elected leaders. Many attend viewings and funerals every week, sharing the grief of mothers and fathers burying their children. These experiences and relationships are opportunities to bring addiction out of the shadows. Confronting stigma can help people at risk feel comfortable asking for help.

What can states do?

In January 2014, Vermont Governor Peter Shumlin devoted his State of the State address to the issue of opioid addiction. He said, "The time has come for us to stop quietly averting our eyes from the growing heroin addiction in our front yards, while we fear and fight treatment facilities in our backyards."[4] Three years later, Ohio Governor John Kasich told his state, "Addiction is an enemy that knows no distinction between incomes or neighborhoods or skin color. Addiction simply seeks to devour everyone and everything. Therefore, there can be no divisions among us as we face this common enemy."[5]

In the last several years, many state leaders, both Democratic and Republican, have been outspoken about the devastation caused by the opioid epidemic. This reckoning is a positive sign, because states have opportunities to develop and implement focused strategies to save lives. As part of these strategies:

States can promote the appropriate care of pain

To prevent addiction from developing, a number of states have pushed the medical profession to prescribe opioids more responsibly. In some places, this effort has taken the shape of new state laws that limit extended prescriptions for new patients. In others, states have required doctors, nurse practitioners, and physician assistants to receive additional education in pain management as a condition of licensure.

In general, these have been steps in the right direction. However, in some places, there is concern that aggressive steps to limit opioid prescribing have frightened doctors from prescribing needed therapy and have led to dangerous interruptions in care for stable patients with chronic pain. State medical boards have a special responsibility to provide guidance (and confidence) to clinicians both about what is not acceptable practice—and what is.

States can expand Medicaid

Organized and implemented at the state level, the Medicaid program is the most important insurer for addiction treatment services in the United States. An estimated 40% of nonelderly adults with opioid addiction have Medicaid coverage.[6] Expanding this program to all low-income individuals and families, as permitted under the Affordable Care Act, allows states to sustainably fund treatment for millions of people.

Recently, some have claimed that Medicaid expansion may make the opioid epidemic worse, by providing greater access to prescription opioids for pain. A well-designed study in August 2018 found strong evidence against this theory. Comparing counties with and without Medicaid expansion, researchers discovered that the expansion was not associated with a greater number of prescriptions for opioid medications for pain. It was, however, associated with a greater number of buprenorphine prescriptions for treatment.[7] In Ohio, speaking of the opioid epidemic Governor Kasich said, "Thank God we expanded Medicaid."[8]

States can create robust systems of care

Beyond reimbursing for addiction treatment, states can assure that high-quality services are available for people when they are most needed.[9] States can direct funding to centers of excellence in addiction treatment that provide rapid access to medication therapy and counseling. These can be paired with recovery services that offer ongoing access to peers and other supports. State Medicaid programs can create incentives for high quality care, such as by providing enhanced payment to providers that adhere to evidence and have successful outcomes. States can also establish strong regulations to stop inappropriate and counterproductive treatment practices.

States can ask for more from their healthcare systems

This effort can include supporting primary care clinicians in offering opioid addiction treatment in their practices, while helping specialty addiction treatment programs provide care for other medical and psychiatric conditions.

There are also opportunities to ask hospitals and health systems to rise to the challenge of the opioid epidemic. In Rhode Island, after the son of a prominent businessman died of an overdose, it was revealed that the young man had visited emergency departments multiple times for nonfatal overdoses in recent weeks. Yet he was never provided treatment or linked to care.[10] The state's health commissioner responded by establishing standards for hospitals that included having peers work in the emergency department and starting treatment as quickly as possible with buprenorphine.[11]

States can fix their correctional systems

There is substantial evidence that detention, parole, and probation are major opportunities to provide effective treatment and, as a result, both save lives and reduce recidivism.[12,13] Unfortunately, because of misunderstanding, lack of resources, and stigma, most of these opportunities are squandered.[14]

The good news is that states are starting to rethink their approaches. For example, in 2015, experts from Brown University recommended to Rhode Island Governor Gina Raimondo that the state provide access to all FDA-approved medications in the state's jail and prison and continue treatment in the community after release.[15] Three years later, after the state funded and implemented this recommendation, researchers reported a 60% decline in fatal overdoses among those leaving detention.[16]

States can repurpose monitoring programs into assistance programs for people with addiction

Many states now require clinicians to check a prescription database, known as a prescription drug monitoring program, to find out if their patients have been receiving opioids from multiple healthcare providers at once, a sign of potential misuse. However, states generally do not provide training and resources to help clinicians care for these patients when a problem is discovered. Doing so would prevent people from leaving a doctor's office empty-handed and searching for opioids on the street.

States can fund harm reduction approaches that are based on evidence

States can make naloxone more widely available, support syringe services programs, permit innovation with new technology such as fentanyl checking, and consider allowing localities to establish overdose prevention sites (with appropriate monitoring and evaluation). Close tracking of these programs can provide data to demonstrate their value to the public.

States can use data to inform their response

States including Rhode Island, California, and Illinois have set up public dashboards to monitor the opioid epidemic and the success of key initiatives. The best of these dashboards keep the focus on whether the crisis is getting better or worse, as measured by real outcomes including fatal and nonfatal overdose.

A few states are going further by developing comprehensive databases to guide future policy. For example, a new Massachusetts law called Chapter 55 allowed the state to merge data sets from hospitals, coroners, and the correctional system related to the opioid crisis.[17] Reports based on this database have found that people leaving the correctional system face an overdose risk more than 100 times greater than that of the general population. Massachusetts has also studied what happens after a nonfatal overdose: people who receive treatment with methadone or buprenorphine have a much lower risk of dying later from an overdose.[18] These results have led the state to expand efforts to provide access to treatment with medications in the correctional system.[19]

States can confront stigma

Many advocates credit Governor Shumlin for using his 2014 State of the State address to treat the opioid epidemic as a crisis affecting families across Vermont—families who "know too well the crushing hurt and harm that comes from opiate addiction."[20] He compared addiction to other chronic illnesses such as diabetes and epilepsy. And he pointed out the connection between addiction and underlying social deprivation, including the lack of educational and employment opportunities. Governor Shumlin's speech was important for its details, but extraordinary for its message: We need to help, not punish, people who are experiencing an addiction.

What can the federal government do?

The federal government can lead the country in applying urgency, evidence, and resources to counter the opioid epidemic.

Urgency is more than declaring an emergency. It requires acting like there is an emergency. Impactful steps can include:

- The Office of National Drug Control Policy in the White House can establish a national dashboard on overdose with reliable and up-to-date data from across the country.
- Within the Department of Health and Human Services (HHS), the FDA can use its authority to identify prescribers of fentanyl and other particularly dangerous opioids who are practicing outside the standard of care and, if other measures fail, stop them from placing patients at

risk. The Secretary of HHS can set a standard for insurers for coverage of non-pharmaceutical approaches to pain.

- The White House can take steps to make naloxone more widely available at lower prices. This can involve a national purchase of naloxone for the public sector, across the Veterans Administration, the Department of Defense, the Centers for Medicare and Medicaid Services, Indian Health Service, and state and local governments. This purchase can be modeled after the federal purchase of vaccines under the Vaccines for Children program. Alternative approaches to obtaining naloxone at lower prices are also available.

- The Attorney General can require that all physicians receive training in appropriate management of pain and in the use of buprenorphine for addiction treatment as a condition of receiving a license to prescribe controlled medications.

- The Drug Enforcement Administration can revisit the regulations on methadone to permit innovations in access to care (such as permitting dispensing in pharmacies), as long as they are well justified, supervised, and evaluated.

- The HHS Secretary can deploy the doctors and nurse practitioners of the US Public Health Service Commissioned Corps to areas of rising overdose across the country to provide rapid access to addiction treatment with buprenorphine and train local providers to continue care. The Commissioned Corps can also be deployed to assist with the care of patients affected when physicians lose their licenses to prescribe controlled medications.

- The Centers for Disease Control and Prevention and the Substance Abuse and Mental Health Services Administration can encourage communities to adopt innovative approaches to the overdose crisis based on evidence, such as offering treatment in syringe services programs and other community locations, implementing fentanyl checking, and establishing overdose prevention sites that offer ready access to treatment. The agencies

can assist with implementation, monitoring, and evaluation of these efforts.

Applying evidence to the opioid epidemic means doing
less of what is counterproductive and more of what saves
lives. The Justice Department can reject calls to escalate the
war on drugs—and instead support access to all three FDA-
approved medications for opioid addiction across the criminal justice system. The Centers for Medicare and Medicaid
Services within HHS can stop states from restricting access to
evidence-based treatment for opioid addiction in the Medicaid
program—while rapidly implementing access to treatment
with methadone within the Medicare program. The federal
government can ask expert organizations, such as the National
Academies of Science, Engineering, and Medicine to identify
areas where federal policy is making matters worse—and to
recommend alternative approaches.

Congress has allocated several billion dollars over the next
few years to address the opioid epidemic, a small fraction of
what is needed. Much more in the ballpark is what Senator
Elizabeth Warren and Congressman Elijah Cummings have
proposed, modeled on the successful Ryan White Care Act for
HIV/AIDS: $100 billion over the next decade.[21] Critical federal
investments are needed to support training, treatment, and
research.

The president of the United States has a role to play too.
Instead of praising dictators who are known for violent
crackdowns on illicit drug use,[22] he can celebrate heroes on the
front lines of the crisis whose committed work is saving lives.
In addition to diplomacy to reduce the production of fentanyl
abroad, the president can make it clear that individuals with
opioid addiction are Americans in need of assistance. He can
assure that the opioid epidemic is met with a public health response. In the words of George Shultz, the Secretary of State
under President Ronald Reagan, and Pedro Aspe, the former
secretary of finance in Mexico, the president can recognize

that the opioid epidemic is not "simply a law enforcement problem, solvable through arrests, prosecution and restrictions on supply" and instead " attack it with public health policies and education."[23]

What can individuals and families do?

All concerned about the opioid epidemic can push their local healthcare system, local police department, local and state government, and national leadership to do better. The voices of individuals and families who have been affected directly by opioids are especially needed. Their engagement requires resisting the urge to hide, fighting the temptation to blame, and rejecting the stigma associated with addiction and its treatment. A first step is to join one of several grassroots organizations lobbying for greater attention to and resources for the opioid epidemic, some of which are listed in Appendix 6.

In the United States, there is a deep commitment to personal responsibility. Consistent with this value, there are steps that each person with addiction can take. But as the U.S. Surgeon General recently noted, the choices people make are 100% dependent on the choices they have in front of them. It is hard to ask someone to reduce the use of opioids for an injury when physical therapy and other alternative services are not available. It is difficult to expect someone to seek care when no effective treatment is accessible or when the only treatment that is available would make things worse. It is essentially impossible to urge someone to find housing or a job when landlords and employers block anyone with a history of drug use.

Citizens can arm themselves with facts and evidence and then speak up and speak out—at local zoning board meetings, town hall gatherings, city and county council sessions, and state and federal hearings. In America, change comes when people demand it. Collectively, the nation can move beyond a state of confusion on opioids to make enduring progress.

Appendix 1

DEFINITIONS OF ADDICTION

American Society of Addiction Medicine

Addiction is a primary, chronic disease of brain reward, motivation, memory and related circuitry. Dysfunction in these circuits leads to characteristic biological, psychological, social and spiritual manifestations. This is reflected in an individual pathologically pursuing reward and/or relief by substance use and other behaviors.

Addiction is characterized by inability to consistently abstain, impairment in behavioral control, craving, diminished recognition of significant problems with one's behaviors and interpersonal relationships, and a dysfunctional emotional response. Like other chronic diseases, addiction often involves cycles of relapse and remission. Without treatment or engagement in recovery activities, addiction is progressive and can result in disability or premature death.

Source: American Society of Addiction Medicine. Definition of Addiction. https://www.asam.org/quality-practice/definition-of-addiction. Accessed October 7, 2018.

Surgeon General of the United States

Addiction: Common name for a severe substance use disorder, associated with compulsive or uncontrolled use of one or more substances. Addiction is a chronic brain disease that has the potential for both recurrence (relapse) and recovery.

Source: US Department of Health and Human Services (HHS), Office of the Surgeon General, *Facing Addiction in America: The Surgeon General's Spotlight on Opioids.* Washington, DC: HHS, September 2018. https://addiction.surgeongeneral.gov/sites/default/files/OC_SpotlightOnOpioids.pdf. Accessed October 7, 2018.

National Institute on Drug Abuse

Addiction is defined as a chronic, relapsing disorder characterized by compulsive drug seeking and use despite adverse consequences. It is considered a brain disorder, because it involves functional changes to brain circuits involved in reward, stress, and self-control, and those changes may last a long time after a person has stopped taking drugs. Addiction is a lot like other diseases, such as heart disease. Both disrupt the normal, healthy functioning of an organ in the body, both have serious harmful effects, and both are, in many cases, preventable and treatable. If left untreated, they can last a lifetime and may lead to death.

Source: National Institute on Drug Abuse. Drugs, brains and behavior: the science of addiction. July 2018. https://www.drugabuse.gov/publications/drugs-brains-behavior-science-addiction/drug-misuse-addiction#footnote. Accessed October 7, 2018.

Appendix 2

NON-STIGMATIZING PREFERRED LANGUAGE

Instead of	Try this non-judgmental alternative
Abstinence-based or abstinence-only	Not including a medication
Addict	Person with a substance use disorder; or person with a serious substance use disorder
Alcoholic	Person with an alcohol use disorder; or person with a serious alcohol use disorder
Clean	Abstinent; or abstaining from
Clean (urine test)	Negative for substance X; or as expected
Consumer/client/patient	Person; or individual; or participant
Dirty	Actively using; or positive for substance use
Dirty (urine test)	Positive for substance X; or unexpected
Drug-free	Not including a medication
Drug habit	Substance use disorder; or compulsive or regular substance use
Drug abuse or substance abuser	Person with a substance use disorder; or person who uses substances (if does not qualify for a diagnosis of substance use disorder)
Enabling	Working with

Instead of	Try this non-judgmental alternative
Former/reformed addict/ alcoholic	Person in remission or recovery; or person in sustained remission or long-term recovery
Graduated	Stabilized
Mentally ill	Person with a mental health disorder
Methadone clinic	Opioid treatment program (OTP)
Non-compliant	Use descriptive terms geared towards stage of change (e.g.: thinking about quitting use)
Not ready	Use descriptive terms geared towards stage of change (e.g.: thinking about quitting use)
Opioid replacement or opioid substitution therapy	Treatment that includes a medication/ treatment with X (name of medication)
Recreational, casual, or experimental users (as opposed to those with a substance use disorder)	People who use drugs for non-medical reasons; or people starting to use drugs; or people who are new to drug use
Self-help	Self-directed; or mutual aid
Sober	Well; or healthy
Substance abuse	Substance use disorder

Sources: Botticelli MP, Koh HK. Changing the language of addiction. *JAMA*. 2016 Oct 4;316(13):1361–1362; Olsen Y. To address addiction, start with words. *Huffington Post.* 21 June 2015. https://www.huffpost.com/entry/addiction-language_b_7097396. Accessed October 7, 2018.

Appendix 3

DEFINITIONS OF RECOVERY

Substance Abuse and Mental Health Services Administration

A process of change through which individuals improve their health and wellness, live self-directed lives, and strive to reach their full potential.

Source: Substance Abuse and Mental Health Services Administration. Recovery and recovery support. 20 September 2017. https://www.samhsa.gov/recovery. Accessed October 7, 2018.

American Society of Addiction Medicine

A process of sustained action that addresses the biological, psychological, social and spiritual disturbances inherent in addiction. Recovery aims to improve the quality of life by seeking balance and healing in all aspects of health and wellness, while addressing an individual's consistent pursuit of abstinence, impairment in behavioral control, dealing with cravings, recognizing problems in one's behaviors and interpersonal relationships, and dealing more effectively with emotional responses.

Source: American Society of Addiction Medicine. Terminology related to addiction, treatment and recovery. July 2013. https://www.asam.org/docs/default-source/public-policy-statements/1-terminology-atr-7-135f81099472bc604ca5b7ff000030b21a.pdf?sfvrsn=d23d69c2_0. Accessed October 7, 2018.

Appendix 4

EXAMPLES OF PHARMACEUTICAL OPIOIDS AVAILABLE IN THE UNITED STATES, DECEMBER 2018

Opioids Used for Pain		
Generic name	Trade names	Formulations
Buprenorphine	Belbuca Buprenex	Buccal film Injection (IV, IM)
	Butrans	Transdermal patch
Butorphanol	—	Injection (IV, IM), Nasal spray
Codeine	—	Tablet, oral solution, injection (SQ, IM)
Codeine/ acetaminophen	Tylenol with Codeine	Tablet
Dihydrocodeine/ acetaminophen/ caffeine	Trezix	Tablet, Capsule

Opioids Used for Pain

Generic name	Trade names	Formulations
Fentanyl	—	Tablet, lozenge, transdermal patch, injection (IV, IM)
	Abstral	Sublingual tablet
	Actiq	Oral transmucosal lozenge
	Duragesic	Transdermal patch
	Fentora	Buccal tablet
	Lazanda	Nasal spray
	Sublimaze	Injection (IV, IM)
	Subsys	Sublingual spray
Hydrocodone	—	Capsule, tablet, oral solution, tablet
	Hysingla ER	Extended-release tablet
	Zohydro ER	Extended-release capsule
Hydrocodone/ acetaminophen	—	Tablet, solution, syrup, elixir, , liquid
	Anexsia	Tablet
	Apadaz	Tablet
	Lortab	Tablet, oral solution
	Norco	Tablet
	Vicodin	Tablet
Hydrocodone/ ibuprofen	—	Tablet
	Reprexain	Tablet
Hydromorphone	—	Tablet, extended-release tablet, injection (IV, IM, SQ)
	Dilaudid	Injection (IV, IM, SQ)
	Exalgo	Extended-release tablet
Levorphanol	—	Tablet
Meperidine	Demerol	Tablet, oral solution, injection (IV, IM)
Methadone	—	Tablet (5 mg and 10 mg only)
	Dolophine	Tablet (5 mg and 10 mg only)
	Methadose	Tablet (10 mg only)

Opioids Used for Pain

Generic name	Trade names	Formulations
Morphine	—	Tablet, capsule, injection (IV, IM, SQ), oral solution, suppositories, extended-release tablets and capsules
	Astramorph-PF	Injection (IV, epidural, intrathecal)
	Duramorph	Injection (IV, epidural, intrathecal)
	Infumorph	Infusion (epidural, intrathecal)
	Kadian	Extended-release capsule
	Morphabond ER	Extended-release tablet
	MS Contin	Controlled-release tablet
Oxycodone	—	Tablet, capsule, solution
	Oxaydo	Tablet
	Oxycontin	Extended-release tablet
	Oxy IR	Tablet
	Roxicodone	Tablet
	Xtampza	Extended-release capsule
Oxycodone/ acetaminophen	—	Tablet
	Endocet	Tablet
	Oxycet	Tablet
	Percocet	Tablet
	Perloxx	Tablet
	Roxicet	Tablet, oral solution
Oxycodone/aspirin	—	Tablet
	Percodan	Tablet
Oxycodone/ ibuprofen	—	Tablet
Oxymorphone	—	Tablet, extended release tablets
	Opana	Tablet
Sufentanil	—	Injection (IV, epidural)
	Dsuvia	Sublingual tablet
	Sufenta	Injection (IV, epidural)

Opioids Used for Pain

Generic name	Trade names	Formulations
Tapentadol	Nucynta	Tablet
	Nucynta ER	Extended release
Tramadol	Conzip	Extended-release capsule
	Ultram	Tablet
Tramadol/ acetaminophen	Ultracet	Tablet

Opioids Used for Opioid Addiction Treatment

Buprenorphine	—	Sublingual tablet
	Probuphine	Implant for subdermal administration
	Sublocade	Injection (SQ), extended release
Buprenorphine/ naloxone	—	Sublingual tablet
	Bunavail	Buccal film
	Cassipa	Sublingual film
	Suboxone	Sublingual film
	Zubsolv	Sublingual tablet
Methadone	—	Tablets, concentrate, oral solution, extended-release Capsules and tablets
	Dolophine	Tablet
	Methadose	Tablet, oral concentrate

Sources: US Food and Drug Administration. List of extended-release and long-acting opioid products required to have an opioid REMS. 24 November 2017. https://www.fda.gov/Drugs/DrugSafety/InformationbyDrugClass/ucm251735.htm. Accessed October 7, 2018. Executive Office of Health and Human Services, Commonwealth of Massachusetts. Table 8: Opioids and analgesics. 10 September 2018. https://masshealthdruglist.ehs.state.ma.us/MHDL/pubtheradetail.do?id=8. Accessed October 7, 2018. U.S. US Food and Drug Administration. Information about medication-assisted treatment (MAT). 3 October 2018. https://www.fda.gov/Drugs/DrugSafety/InformationbyDrugClass/ucm600092.htm. Accessed October 7, 2018.

US Food and Drug Administration. Drugs@FDA database. Accessed December 10, 2018.

Appendix 5

DIAGNOSTIC CRITERIA
FOR OPIOID USE DISORDER

A problematic pattern of opioid use leading to clinically significant impairment or distress, as manifested by at least two of the following, occurring within a 12-month period:

1. Opioids are often taken in larger amounts or over a longer period than was intended.
2. There is a persistent desire or unsuccessful efforts to cut down or control opioid use.
3. A great deal of time is spent in activities necessary to obtain the opioid, use the opioid, or recover from its effects.
4. Craving, or a strong desire or urge to use opioids.
5. Recurrent opioid use resulting in a failure to fulfill major role obligations at work, school, or home.
6. Continued opioid use despite having persistent or recurrent social or interpersonal problems caused or exacerbated by the effects of opioids.
7. Important social, occupational, or recreational activities are given up or reduced because of opioid use.
8. Recurrent opioid use in situations in which it is physically hazardous.
9. Continued opioid use despite knowledge of having a persistent or recurrent physical or psychological problem

that is likely to have been caused or exacerbated by the substance.

10. Tolerance, as defined by either of the following:
    a. A need for markedly increased amounts of opioids to achieve intoxication or desired effect.
    b. A markedly diminished effect with continued use of the same amount of an opioid.
       - **Note:** This criterion is not considered to be met for those taking opioids solely under appropriate medical supervision.

11. Withdrawal, as manifested by either of the following:
    a. The characteristic opioid withdrawal syndrome (refer to Criteria A and B of the criteria set for opioid withdrawal, pp. 547–548).
    b. Opioids (or a closely related substance) are taken to relieve or avoid withdrawal symptoms.
       - **Note:** This criterion is not considered to be met for those individuals taking opioids solely under appropriate medical supervision.

Mild opioid use disorder is indicated by the presence of 2 to 3 symptoms; moderate, 4 to 5 symptoms; and severe, 6 or more symptoms.

Source: American Psychiatric Association. *Diagnostic and statistical manual of mental disorders (DSM-5).* 5th ed. Washington, DC: American Psychiatric Publishing, 2013.

Appendix 6

RECOVERY ORGANIZATIONS
(Listed in alphabetical order)

Addiction Policy Forum https://www.addictionpolicy.org/

Faces and Voices of Recovery https://facesandvoicesofrecovery.org/

Facing Addiction with NCADD https://www.facingaddiction.org/

M.A.R.S. Project http://marsproject.org/

National Council on Alcoholism and Drug Dependence https://www.ncadd.org/

National Council on Behavioral Health https://www.thenationalcouncil.org/

Shatterproof https://www.shatterproof.org/

NOTES

Chapter 1

1. Cannabis, coca, & poppy: nature's addictive plants. *DEA Museum.* https://www.deamuseum.org/ccp/opium/history. html. Accessed August 27, 2018.
2. Turkey top opium producer. *Hurriyet Daily News.* 20 November 2012. https://www.deamuseum.org/ccp/opium/history.html. Accessed August 27, 2018.
3. Booth M. *Opium: A History.* New York, NY: Simon & Shuster; 1996.
4. Merrall EL, Kariminia A, Binswanger IA, Hobbs MS, Farrell M, Marsden J, Hutchinson SJ, Bird SM. Meta-analysis of drug-related deaths soon after release from prison. *Addiction.* 2010 Sep;105(9):1545–1554.
5. Lurie J. Go to jail, die from drug withdrawal: welcome to the criminal justice system. *Mother Jones.* 5 February 2017. https://www.motherjones.com/politics/2017/02/opioid-withdrawal-jail-deaths/. Accessed August 12, 2018.
6. Martin WR, Jasinski DR. Physiological parameters of morphine dependence in man—tolerance, early abstinence, protracted abstinence. *J Psychiatr Res.* 1969;7(1):9–17.
7. Volkow ND, Koob GF, McLellan AT. Neurobiologic advances from the brain disease model of addiction. *N Engl J Med.* 2016;374(4):363–371.
8. Barry CL, McGinty EE, Pescosolido BA, Goldman HH. Stigma, discrimination, treatment effectiveness, and policy: public

views about drug addiction and mental illness. *Psychiatr Serv.* 2014;65(10):1269–1272.

9. Kelly JF, Westerhoff CM. Does it matter how we refer to individuals with substance-related conditions? A randomized study of two commonly used terms. *Int J Drug Policy.* 2010 May;21(3):202–207.

10. White House Office of the National Drug Control Policy. *Changing the Language of Addiction.* 9 January 2017. https://www.whitehouse.gov/sites/whitehouse.gov/files/images/Memo%20-%20Changing%20Federal%20Terminology%20Regrading%20Substance%20Use%20and%20Substance%20Use%20Disorders.pdf. Accessed August 27, 2018.

11. Christensen P. Style guide changes address language about addiction, gender. *Association of Health Care Journalists.* 21 June 2017. https://healthjournalism.org/blog/2017/06/style-guide-changes-address-language-about-addiction-gender/. Accessed August 27, 2018.

12. Musto DF. *The American Disease: Origins of Narcotic Control.* 3rd edition. New York: Oxford University Press; 1999.

13. FTC, FDA warn companies about marketing and selling opioid cessation products. *Federal Trade Commission.* 24 January 2018. https://www.ftc.gov/news-events/press-releases/2018/01/ftc-fda-warn-companies-about-marketing-selling-opioid-cessation. Accessed August 25, 2018.

14. Robins LN, Davis DH, Goodwin DW. Drug use by U.S. Army enlisted men in Vietnam: a follow-up on their return home. *Am J Epidemiol.* 1974;99(4):235–249.

15. McLellan AT, Arndt IO, Metzger DS, Woody GE, O'Brien CP. The effects of psychosocial services in substance abuse treatment. *JAMA.* 1993;269(15):1953–1959.

16. Mattick RP, Breen C, Kimber J, Davoli M. Buprenorphine maintenance versus placebo or methadone maintenance for opioid dependence. *Cochrane Database Syst Rev.* 2014;(2):CD002207.

17. Clausen T, Anchersen K, Waal H. Mortality prior to, during and after opioid maintenance treatment (OMT): a national prospective cross-registry study. *Drug Alcohol Depend.* 2008;94(1–3):151–157.

18. Low AJ, Mburu G, Welton NJ, et al. Impact of opioid substitution therapy on antiretroviral therapy outcomes: a systematic review and meta-analysis. *Clin Infect Dis.* 2016;63(8):1094–1104.

19. Nielsen S, Larance B, Degenhardt L, Gowing L, Kehler C, Lintzeris N. Opioid agonist treatment for pharmaceutical opioid dependent people. *Cochrane Database Syst Rev.* 2016;(5):CD011117.

20. Schwartz RP, Gryczynski J, O'Grady KE, et al. Opioid agonist treatments and heroin overdose deaths in Baltimore, Maryland, 1995–2009. *Am J Public Health.* 2013;103(5):917–922.

21. Krupitsky E, Nunes EV, Ling W, Illeperuma A, Gastfriend DR, Silverman BL. Injectable extended-release naltrexone for opioid dependence: a double-blind, placebo-controlled, multicentre randomised trial. *Lancet.* 2011;377(9776):1506–1513.

22. May K. Recovering addict says Walgreens pharmacist denied to fill Rx that helps her stay sober. *Fox 45.* 19 September 2017. https://fox45now.com/news/local/recovering-addict-says-walgreens-pharmacist-denied-to-fill-rx-that-helps-her-stay-sober. Accessed August 30, 2018.

23. Remarks from FDA Commissioner Scott Gottlieb, M.D., as prepared for oral testimony before the House Committee on Energy and Commerce Hearing, "Federal Efforts to Combat the Opioid Crisis: A Status Update on CARA and Other Initiatives. *U.S. Food and Drug Administration.* 25 October 2017. https://www.fda.gov/NewsEvents/Newsroom/PressAnnouncements/ucm582031.htm. Accessed August 27, 2018.

24. National Institutes of Health. *Drugs, Brains, and Behavior: The Science of Addiction.* July 2018. https://www.drugabuse.gov/publications/drugs-brains-behavior-science-addiction/treatment-recovery. Accessed September 30, 2018.

25. Ashford RD, Brown AM, Curtis B. Substance use, recovery, and linguistics: the impact of word choice on explicit and implicit bias. *Drug Alcohol Depend.* 2018 Aug 1;189:131–138.

26. Armstrong D. 52 weeks, 52 faces. *Stat News.* 20 December 2016. https://www.statnews.com/feature/opioid-epidemic/obituaries/. Accessed August 9, 2018.

27. Seven days of heroin. *The Cincinnati Enquirer.* 10 September 2017. https://www.cincinnati.com/pages/interactives/seven-days-of-heroin-epidemic-cincinnati/. Accessed August 10, 2018.

28. Nachtwey J. The Opioid Diaries. *TIME.* 5 March 2018.

29. Substance Abuse and Mental Health Services Administration. *Key Substance Use and Mental Health Indicators in the United States: Results from the 2016 National Survey on Drug Use and Health* (HHS Publication No. SMA 17-5044, NSDUH Series H-52).

2017. Rockville, MD: Center for Behavioral Health Statistics and Quality, Substance Abuse and Mental Health Services Administration.

30. Quast T, Storch EA, Yampolskaya S. Opioid prescription rates and child removals: evidence from Florida. *Health Aff.* 2018;37(1):134–139.

31. Noguchi Y. Opioid crisis looms over job market, worrying employers and economists. *NPR.* 7 September 2017. https://www.npr.org/2017/09/07/545602212/opioid-crisis-looms-over-job-market-worrying-employers-and-economists. Accessed August 27, 2018.

32. The Council of Economic Advisors. *The Underestimated Cost of the Opioid Crisis.* November 2017. https://www.whitehouse.gov/sites/whitehouse.gov/files/images/The%20Underestimated%20Cost%20of%20the%20Opioid%20Crisis.pdf. Accessed August 25, 2018.

33. Goodnough A. Injecting drugs can ruin a heart: how many second chances should a user get? *The New York Times.* 29 April 2018.

34. Bebinger M. Black drug users grapple with surging opioid overdose death rates. *WBUR.* 24 May 2018. http://www.wbur.org/commonhealth/2018/05/24/blacks-dying-more-from-opioid-overdoses-than-whites. Accessed August 27, 2018.

35. Gomes T, Tadrous M, Mamdani M, et al. The burden of opioid-related mortality in the United States. *JAMA Network Open.* 2018;1(2):e180217.

36. Nachtwey J. The Opioid Diaries. *TIME.* 5 March 2018.

37. Bernstein L. U.S. life expectancy declines again, a dismal trend not seen since World War I. The Washington Post. 29 November 2018. https://www.washingtonpost.com/national/health-science/us-life-expectancy-declines-again-a-dismal-trend-not-seen-since-world-war-i/2018/11/28/ae58bc8c-f28c-11e8-bc79-68604ed88993_story.html?utm_term=.180bb0633195. Accessed December 8, 2018.

38. Centers for Disease Control and Prevention. *The Public Health System & the 10 Essential Public Health Services.* 26 June 2018. https://www.cdc.gov/stltpublichealth/publichealthservices/essentialhealthservices.html. Accessed August 25, 2018.

39. Goodnough A. This city's overdose deaths have plunged. Can others learn from it? The New York Times. 25 November 2018. https://www.nytimes.com/2018/11/25/health/opioid-overdose-deaths-dayton.html. Accessed December 8, 2018.

40. Sharfstein JM. A new year's wish on opioids. *JAMA*. 2018;319(6):537.

Chapter 2

1. Goldstein L, Lymberopoulous G. Changing opioid prescribing patterns for post-extraction dental pain. *Practical Pain Management*. 9 May 2017. https://www.practicalpainmanagement.com/resources/news-and-research/changing-opioid-prescribing-patterns-post-extraction-dental-pain. Accessed August 27, 2018.

2. Yi P, Pryzbylkowski P. Opioid induced hyperalgesia. *Pain Med*. 2015;16(suppl 1):S32–S36.

3. Krebs EE, Gravely A, Nugent S, et al. Effect of opioid vs nonopioid medications on pain-related function in patients with chronic back pain or hip or knee osteoarthritis pain: the SPACE randomized clinical trial. *JAMA*. 2018;319(9):872–882.

4. Massachusetts Executive Office of Health and Human Services. Table 8: opioids and analgesics. 30 July 2018. https://masshealthdruglist.ehs.state.ma.us/MHDL/pubtheradetail.do?id=8. Accessed August 29, 2018.

5. FDA drug safety communication: FDA warns about serious risks and death when combining opioid pain or cough medicines with benzodiazepines; requires its strongest warning. *U.S. Food and Drugs Administration*. 20 September 2017. https://www.fda.gov/drugs/drugsafety/ucm518473.htm. Accessed August 25, 2018.

6. Pernia S, DeMaagd G. The new pregnancy and lactation labeling rule. *Pharm Ther*. 2016;41(11):713–715.

7. Yi P, Pryzbylkowski P. Opioid induced hyperalgesia. *Pain Med*. 2015;16(suppl 1):S32–S36.

8. Plein LM, Rittner HL. Opioids and the immune system—friend or foe. *Br J Pharmacol*. 2018;175(14):2717–2725.

9. Maruta T, Swanson DW, Finlayson RE. Drug abuse and dependency in patients with chronic pain. *Mayo Clin Proc*. 1976;54:241–244.

10. Evans PJD. Narcotic addiction in patients with chronic pain. *Anesthesia*. 1981;36:597–602.

11. Fishbain DA, Rosomoff HL, Rosomoff RS. Drug abuse, dependence and addiction in chronic pain patients. *Clin J Pain.* 1992;8:77–85.

12. Kouyanou K, Pither C, Wessely S. Medication misuse, abuse and dependence in chronic pain patients. *J Psychosomatic Res.* 1997;43:497–504.

13. Vowles KE, McEntee ML, Julnes PS, Frohe T, Ney JP, van der Goes DN. Rates of opioid misuse, abuse, and addiction in chronic pain: a systematic review and data synthesis. *Pain.* 2015;156(4):569–576.

14. Shah A, Hayes CJ, Martin BC. Characteristics of initial prescription episodes and likelihood of long-term opioid use—United States, 2006–2015. *MMWR Morb Mortal Wkly Rep.* 2017;66(10):265–269.

15. Krebs EE, Lorenz KA, Bair MJ, et al. Development and initial validation of the PEG, a three-item scale assessing pain intensity and interference. *J Gen Intern Med.* 2009;24(6):733–738.

16. Chiarotto A, Maxwell LJ, Ostelo RW, Boers M, Tugwell P, Terwee CB. Measurement properties of visual analogue scale, numeric rating scale and pain severity subscale of the brief pain inventory in patients with low back pain: a systematic review. *J Pain.* 2018. https://doi.org/10.1016/j.jpain.2018.07.009

17. Centers for Disease Control and Prevention. *Pocket Guide: Tapering Opioids for Chronic Pain.* August 2017. https://www.cdc.gov/drugoverdose/pdf/clinical_pocket_guide_tapering-a.pdf. Accessed August 27, 2018.

18. American Medical Association. *Help Save Lives: Co-Prescribe Naloxone to Patients at Risk of Overdose.* August 2017. https://www.end-opioid-epidemic.org/wp-content/uploads/2017/08/AMA-Opioid-Task-Force-naloxone-one-pager-updated-August-2017-FINAL.pdf. Accessed August 27, 2018.

19. Dowell D, Haegerich TM, Chou R. CDC guideline for prescribing opioids for chronic pain—United States, 2016. *MMWR Recomm Rep.* 2016;65(No. RR-1):1–49.

20. Get trained to administer naloxone and save a life from opioid overdose. *Don't Die.* http://dontdie.org/. Accessed August 27, 2018.

21. Substance Abuse and Mental Health Services Administration. *Key Substance Use and Mental Health Indicators in the United States: Results from the 2016 National Survey on Drug Use and*

Health. September 2017. https://www.samhsa.gov/data/sites/
default/files/NSDUH-FFR1-2016/NSDUH-FFR1-2016.pdf.
Accessed August 29, 2018.

22. US Food and Drugs Administration. *Disposal of unused
medicines: what you should know*. 25 July 2018. https://
www.fda.gov/drugs/resourcesforyou/consumers/
buyingusingmedicinesafely/ensuringsafeuseofmedicine/
safedisposalofmedicines/ucm186187.htm. Accessed August
12, 2018.

23. US Food and Drugs Administration. *Disposal of unused
medicines: what you should know*. 25 July 2018. https://
www.fda.gov/drugs/resourcesforyou/consumers/
buyingusingmedicinesafely/ensuringsafeuseofmedicine/
safedisposalofmedicines/ucm186187.htm. Accessed August
12, 2018.

24. Walmart launches groundbreaking disposal solution to aid in
fight against opioid abuse and misuse. *Walmart*. 17 January 2018.
https://news.walmart.com/2018/01/17/walmart-launches-
groundbreaking-disposal-solution-to-aid-in-fight-against-opioid-
abuse-and misuse. Accessed August 29, 2018.

25. Deterra drug deactivation system. https://deterrasystem.com/.
Accessed August 29, 2018.

Chapter 3

1. Prince died from "exceeding high" amount of fentanyl, experts
say. *USA Today*. 27 March 2018.

2. US Drug Enforcement Administration. *Controlled Substances by
CSA Schedule*. 12 July 2018. https://www.deadiversion.usdoj.
gov/schedules/orangebook/e_cs_sched.pdf. Accessed August
15, 2018.

3. Alambyan V, Pace J, Miller B, et al. The emerging role of inhaled
heroin in the opioid epidemic: A review. *JAMA Neurol*. 2018 Jul
9. http://www.doi.org/10.1001/jamaneurol.2018.1693.

4. Dube SR, Felitti VJ, Dong M, Chapman DP, Giles WH, Anda RF.
Childhood abuse, neglect, and household dysfunction and the
risk of illicit drug use: the adverse childhood experiences study.
Pediatrics. 2003;111(3):564–572.

5. Cicero TJ, Ellis MS, Surratt HL, Kurtz SP. The changing face of
heroin use in the United States: a retrospective analysis of the
past 50 years. *JAMA Psychiatry*. 2014;71(7):821–826.

6. Cicero TJ, Ellis MS, Kasper ZA. Increased use of heroin as an initiating opioid of abuse. Addict Behav. 2017 Nov;74:63–66.

7. Sherman SG, Kamarulzaman A, Spittal P. Women and drugs across the globe: a call to action. *Int J Drug Policy.* 2008;19(2):97–98.

8. Agnich LE, Stogner JM, Miller BL, Marcum CD. Purple drank prevalence and characteristics of misusers of codeine cough syrup mixtures. *Addictive Behaviors.* 2013;38:2445–2449.

9. Ritter A, Cameron J. A review of the efficacy and effectiveness of harm reduction strategies for alcohol, tobacco and illicit drugs. *Drug Alcohol Rev.* 2006 Nov;25(6):611–624.

10. Csete J, Kamarulzaman A, Kazatchkine M, et al. Public health and international drug policy. *Lancet.* 2016 Apr 2;387(10026):1427–1480.

Chapter 4

1. Blum K, Oscar-Berman M, Giordano J, et al. Neurogenetic impairments of brain reward circuitry links to Reward Deficiency Syndrome (RDS): Potential nutrigenomic induced dopaminergic activation. *J Genet Syndr Gene Ther.* 2012;3(4):1000e115.

2. Dube SR, Felitti VJ, Dong M, Chapman DP, Giles WH, Anda RF. Childhood abuse, neglect, and household dysfunction and the risk of illicit drug use: the adverse childhood experiences study. *Pediatrics.* 2003;111(3):564–572.

3. Disease. *Merriam-Webster.* 2018. https://www.merriam-webster.com/dictionary/disease. Accessed August 27, 2018.

4. Perrone M. AP-NORC poll: most Americans see drug addiction as a disease. *U.S. News.* 5 April 2018.

5. American Psychiatric Association. *Diagnostic and Statistical Manual of Mental Disorders.* 5th ed. Arlington, VA: American Psychiatric Association; 2013.

6. Dennis ML, Foss MA, Scott CK. An eight-year perspective on the relationship between the duration of abstinence and other aspects of recovery. *Eval Rev.* 2007;31(6):585–612.

Chapter 5

1. Gudin JA, Mogali S, Jones JD, Comer SD. Risks, management, and monitoring of combination opioid, benzodiazepines, and/or alcohol use. *Postgrad Med.* 2013;125(4):115–130.

2. BLS suspected opioid overdose algorithm. *ACLS Medical Training.* https://www.aclsmedicaltraining.com/

bls-suspected-opioid-overdose-algorithm/. Accessed
September 28, 2018. Basic life support training includes
instruction on when to use rescue breathing and chest
compressions as part of resuscitation in the setting of a
suspected opioid overdose.

3. Faul M, Lurie P, Kinsman JM, Dailey MW, Crabaugh C, Sasser
SM. Multiple naloxone administrations among emergency
medical service providers is increasing. *Prehosp Emerg Care.*
2017;21(4):411–419.

4. Abrams A. The Surgeon General says more people should carry
naloxone, the opioid antidote. Here's where to get it and how
much it costs. *TIME.* 5 April 2018.

5. Narcan nasal spray. *Adapt Pharma.* https://www.narcan.com/
affordability. Accessed August 29, 2018.

6. Doyle R. The limits of charity from a drug company. *The
New Yorker.* 28 February 2017.

7. Maryland Behavioral Health Administration. *Statewide Standing
Order for Pharmacy Naloxone Dispensing.* https://bha.health.
maryland.gov/NALOXONE/Pages/Statewide-Standing-Order.
aspx. Accessed August 29, 2018.

Chapter 6

1. DiClemente CC, Prochaska JO, Fairhurst SK, Velicer
WF, Velasquez MM, Rossi JS. The process of smoking
cessation: an analysis of precontemplation, contemplation,
and preparation stages of change. *J Consult Clin Psychol.*
1991;59(2):295–304.

2. Park-Lee E, Lipari RN, Hedden SL, Kroutil LA, Porter JD; RTI
International. *Receipt of Services for Substance Use and Mental
Health Issues among Adults: Results from the 2016 National Survey on
Drug Use and Health.* 2017. https://www.samhsa.gov/data/sites/
default/files/NSDUH-DR-FFR2-2016/NSDUH-DR-FFR2-2016.
pdf. Accessed August 30, 2018.

3. Cui C, Noronha A, Warren KR, et al. Brain pathways to recovery
from alcohol dependence. *Alcohol.* 2015;49(5):435–452.

4. Substance Abuse and Mental Health Services Administration.
*Medications for Opioid Use Disorder. Treatment Improvement Protocol
(TIP) Series 63, Executive Summary.* February 2018. https://store.
samhsa.gov/shin/content//SMA18-5063EXSUMM/SMA18-
5063EXSUMM.pdf. Accessed August 30, 2018.

5. Dole VP, Nyswander M. A medical treatment for diacetylmorphine (heroin) addiction: a clinical trial with methadone hydrochloride. *JAMA.* 1965;193:646–650.

6. Strain EC, Bigelow GE, Liebson IA, Stitzer ML. Moderate- vs high-dose methadone in the treatment of opioid dependence: a randomized trial. *JAMA.* 1999;281(11):1000–1005.

7. Mattick RP, Breen C, Kimber J, Davoli M. Methadone maintenance therapy versus no opioid replacement therapy for opioid dependence. *Cochrane Database Syst Rev.* 2009;(3):CD002209.

8. Mattick RP, Breen C, Kimber J, Davoli M. Methadone maintenance therapy versus no opioid replacement therapy for opioid dependence. *Cochrane Database Syst Rev.* 2009;(3):CD002209.

9. Rastegar DA, Sharfstein Kawasaki S, King VL, Harris EE, Brooner RK. Criminal charges prior to and after enrollment in opioid agonist treatment: a comparison of methadone maintenance and office-based buprenorphine. *Subst Use Misuse.* 2016;51(7):803–811.

10. Hsiao CY, Chen KC, Lee LT, et al. The reductions in monetary cost and gains in productivity with methadone maintenance treatment: one year follow-up. *Psychiatry Res.* 2015;225(3):673–679.

11. Gowing LR, Farrell M, Bornemann R, Sullivan LE, Ali RL. Brief report: methadone treatment of injecting opioid users for prevention of HIV infection. *J Gen Intern Med.* 2006;21(2):193–195.

12. MacArthur GJ, Minozzi S, Martin N, et al. Opiate substitution treatment and HIV transmission in people who inject drugs: systematic review and meta-analysis. *BMJ.* 2012;345:e5945.

13. Tsui JI, Evans JL, Lum PJ, Hahn JA, Page K. Association of opioid agonist therapy with lower incidence of hepatitis C virus infection in young adult injection drug users. *JAMA Intern Med.* 2014;174(12):1974–1981.

14. Teoh Bing Fei J, Yee A, Habil MH, Danaee M. Effectiveness of methadone maintenance therapy and improvement in quality of life following a decade of implementation. *J Subst Abuse Treat.* 2016;69:50–56.

15. Clausen T, Anchersen K, Waal H. Mortality prior to, during and after opioid maintenance treatment (OMT): a national prospective cross-registry study. *Drug Alcohol Depend.* 2008;94(1-3):151–157.

16. Substance Abuse and Mental Health Services Administration. *Guidelines for Opioid Treatment Programs*. 2015. https://store. samhsa.gov/shin/content/PEP15-FEDGUIDEOTP/PEP15-FEDGUIDEOTP.pdf. Accessed August 29, 2018.

17. Johnson RE, Jaffe JH, Fudala PJ. A controlled trial of buprenorphine treatment for opioid dependence. *JAMA*. 1992;267(20):2750–2755.

18. US Drug Enforcement Administration. *DEA Requirements for DATA Waived Physicians (DWPs)*. https://www.deadiversion. usdoj.gov/pubs/docs/dwp_buprenorphine.htm. Accessed August 29, 2018.

19. Mattick RP, Breen C, Kimber J, Davoli M. Buprenorphine maintenance versus placebo or methadone maintenance for opioid dependence. *Cochrane Database Syst Rev*. 2014;(2):CD002207.

20. Mattick RP, Breen C, Kimber J, Davoli M. Buprenorphine maintenance versus placebo or methadone maintenance for opioid dependence. *Cochrane Database Syst Rev*. 2014;(2):CD002207.

21. Metzger DS, Donnell D, Celentano DD, et al. Expanding substance use treatment options for HIV prevention with buprenorphine-naloxone: HIV Prevention Trials Network 058. *J Acquir Immune Defic Syndr*. 2015;68(5):554–561.

22. Schwartz RP, Gryczynski J, O'Grady KE, et al. Opioid agonist treatments and heroin overdose deaths in Baltimore, Maryland, 1995–2009. *Am J Public Health*. 2013;103(5):917–922.

23. Lee JD, Nunes EV Jr, Novo P, et al. Comparative effectiveness of extended-release naltrexone versus buprenorphine-naloxone for opioid relapse prevention (X:BOT): a multicentre, open-label, randomised controlled trial. *Lancet*. 2018;391(10118):309–318.

24. Larochelle MR, Bernson D, Land T. Medication for opioid use disorder after nonfatal opioid overdose and association with mortality: a cohort study. *Ann Intern Med*. 2018;169(3):137–145.

25. Nosyk B, Sun H, Evans E, et al. Defining dosing pattern characteristics of successful tapers following methadone maintenance treatment: results from a population-based retrospective cohort study. *Addiction*. 2012;107(9):1621–1629.

26. Termorshuizen F, Krol A, Prins M, Geskus R, van den Brink W, van Ameijden EJ. Prediction of relapse to frequent heroin use and the role of methadone prescription: an analysis of the

Amsterdam cohort Study among drug users. *Drug Alcohol Depend*. 2005;79(2):231–240.

27. National Academies of Science, Engineering, and Medicine. *The Health Effects of Cannabis and Cannabinoids: The Current State of Evidence and Recommendations for Research*. 12 January 2017. http://www.nationalacademies.org/hmd/Reports/2017/health-effects-of-cannabis-and-cannabinoids.aspx. Accessed September 1, 2018.

28. Mayo Clinic. Kratom for opioid withdrawal: Does it work? 17 May 2018. https://www.mayoclinic.org/diseases-conditions/prescription-drug-abuse/in-depth/kratom-opioid-withdrawal/art-20402170. Accessed September 1, 2018.

29. Food and Drug Administration. FDA warns companies selling illegal, unapproved kratom products marketed for opioid cessation, pain treatment and other medical uses. 22 May 2018. https://www.fda.gov/NewsEvents/Newsroom/PressAnnouncements/ucm608447.htm. Accessed September 1, 2018.

30. Litjens RP, Brunt TM. How toxic is ibogaine? *Clin Toxicol (Phila)*. 2016;54(4):297–302.

31. Karasz A, Zallman L, Berg K, Gourevitch M, Selwyn P, Arnsten JH. The experience of chronic severe pain in patients undergoing methadone maintenance treatment. *J Pain Symptom Manage*. 2004 Nov;28(5):517–525.

32. FDA. FDA approves the first non-opioid treatment for management of opioid withdrawal symptoms in adults. 16 May 2018. https://www.fda.gov/newsevents/newsroom/pressannouncements/ucm607884.htm. Accessed August 29, 2018.

33. Jarvis M, Williams J, Hurford M, et al. Appropriate use of drug testing in clinical addiction medicine. *J Addict Med*. 2017;11(3):163–173.

Chapter 7

1. Klaman SL, Isaacs K, Leopold A, et al. Treating women who are pregnant and parenting for opioid use disorder and the concurrent care of their infants and children. *J Addict Med*. 2017;11(3):178–190.

2. Jones HE, Terplan M, Meyer M. Medically assisted withdrawal (detoxification): considering the mother–infant dyad. *J Addict Med*. 2017;11(2):90–92.

3. Jones HE, Kaltenbach K, Heil SH, et al. Neonatal abstinence syndrome after methadone or buprenorphine exposure. *N Engl J Med.* 2010;363(24):2320–2331.

4. Ko JY, Wolicki S, Barfield WD, et al. CDC grand rounds: public health strategies to prevent neonatal abstinence syndrome. *MMWR Morb Mortal Wkly Rep.* 2017;66(9):242–245.

5. Kocherlakota P. Neonatal abstinence syndrome. *Pediatrics.* 2014;134(2):e547–e561.

6. Mactier H, McLaughlin P, Gillis C, Osselton MD. Variations in infant CYP2B6 genotype associated with the need for pharmacological treatment for neonatal abstinence syndrome in infants of methadone-maintained opioid-dependent mothers. *Am J Perinatol.* 2017;34(9):918–921.

7. Kraft WK, Adeniyi-Jones SC, Chervoneva I, et al. Buprenorphine for the treatment of the neonatal abstinence syndrome. *N Engl J Med.* 2017;376(24):2341–2348.

8. Davis JM, Shenberger J, Terrin N, et al. Comparison of safety and efficacy of methadone vs morphine for treatment of neonatal abstinence syndrome: A randomized clinical trial. *JAMA Pediatr.* 2018;172(8):741–748.

9. American Academy of Pediatrics. Alternative treatment approach for neonatal abstinence syndrome may shorten hospital stay. *EurekAlert!* 4 May 2017. https://www.eurekalert.org/pub_releases/2017-05/aaop-ata042617.php. Accessed August 27, 2018.

10. Sharfstein J. JAMA Forum: Neonatal Abstinence Syndrome: Deja Vu All Over Again? 21 October 2015. http://newsatjama.jama.com/2015/10/21/neonatal-abstinence-syndrome-deja-vu-all-over-again/. Accessed December 8, 2018.

11. Barol B, Prout L, Fitzgerald K, Katz S, King P. Cocaine babies: hooked at birth. *Newsweek.* 2 July 1986.

12. Langone J. Medicine: crack comes to the nursery. *TIME.* 19 September 1988.

13. Dailard C, Nash E. State responses to substance abuse among pregnant women. *Guttmacher Policy Review.* 1 December 2000.

14. Okie S. The epidemic that wasn't. *The New York Times.* 26 January 2009.

15. Fitzgerald S. "Crack baby" study ends with unexpected but clear result. *Philadelphia Inquirer.* 21 July 2013.

16. Bernstein, L. When life begins in rehab: a baby heals after a mother's heroin addiction. *The Washington Post.* 12 August 2015.

17. Smith T. Drug addicts at birth. *Times Daily.* 12 December 2014. http://www.timesdaily.com/news/drug-addicts-at-birth/article_e0cdd95c-8285-11e4-a107-67d4e6a4ebc2.html. Accessed August 27, 2018.

18. Jansson L. Neonatal abstinence syndrome. *UpToDate.* 27 July 2018. https://www.uptodate.com/contents/neonatal-abstinence-syndrome. Accessed August 27, 2018.

19. Dube SR, Felitti VJ, Dong M, Chapman DP, Giles WH, Anda RF. Childhood abuse, neglect, and household dysfunction and the risk of illicit drug use: the adverse childhood experiences study. *Pediatrics.* 2003;111(3):564–572.

20. Kaltenbach K, O'Grady KE, Heil SH, et al. Prenatal exposure to methadone or buprenorphine: early childhood developmental outcomes. *Drug Alcohol Depend.* 2018;185:40.

21. Normile B, Hanlon C. WV Medicaid covers an innovative and less costly treatment model for opioid-affected infants. *National Academy for State Health Policy.* 27 February 2018. https://nashp.org/wv-medicaid-covers-an-innovative-and-less-costly-treatment-model-for-opioid-affected-infants/. Accessed August 27, 2018.

Chapter 8

1. Committee on Substance Use and Prevention. Medication-assisted treatment of adolescents with opioid use disorders. *Pediatrics.* 2016;138(3).

2. Committee on Substance Use and Prevention. Medication-assisted treatment of adolescents with opioid use disorders. *Pediatrics.* 2016;138(3).

3. Gaither JR, Leventhal JM, Ryan SA, Camenga DR. National trends in hospitalizations for opioid poisonings among children and adolescents, 1997 to 2012. *JAMA Pediatr.* 2016;170(12):1195–1201.

4. Committee on Substance Use and Prevention. Medication-assisted treatment of adolescents with opioid use disorders. *Pediatrics.* 2016;138(3).

5. Wenner A, Gigli KH. Opioid addiction in adolescents: A background and policy brief. *J Pediatr Health Care.* 2016;30(6):606–609.

6. Schepis TS, Krishnan-Sarin S. Sources of prescriptions for misuse by adolescents: differences in sex, ethnicity, and severity of

misuse in a population-based study. *J Am Acad Child Adolesc Psychiatry.* 2009;48(8):828–836.

7. Sharma B, Bruner A, Barnett G, Fishman M. Opioid use disorders. *Child Adolesc Psychiatr Clin N Am.* 2016;25(3):473–487.

8. Sharma B, Bruner A, Barnett G, Fishman M. Opioid use disorders. *Child Adolesc Psychiatr Clin N Am.* 2016;25(3):473–487.

9. Subramaniam GA, Stitzer MA. Clinical characteristics of treatment-seeking prescription opioid vs. heroin-using adolescents with opioid use disorder. *Drug Alcohol Depend.* 2009;101(1–2):13–19.

10. Wu LT, Blazer DG, Li TK, Woody GE. Treatment use and barriers among adolescents with prescription opioid use disorders. *Addict Behav.* 2011;36(12):1233–1239.

11. Schuman-Olivier Z, Claire Greene M, Bergman BG, Kelly JF. Is residential treatment effective for opioid use disorders? A longitudinal comparison of treatment outcomes among opioid dependent, opioid misusing, and non-opioid using emerging adults with substance use disorder. *Drug Alcohol Depend.* 2014;144:178–185.

12. Marsch LA, Bickel WK, Badger GJ, et al. Comparison of pharmacological treatments for opioid-dependent adolescents: a randomized controlled trial. *Arch Gen Psychiatry.* 2005;62(10):1157–1164.

13. Woody GE, Poole SA, Subramaniam G, et al. Extended vs short-term buprenorphine-naloxone for treatment of opioid-addicted youth: a randomized trial. *JAMA.* 2008;300(17):2003–2011. Erratum in: *JAMA.* 2009;301(8):830. *JAMA.* 2013;309(14):1461.

14. Knudsen HK, Abraham AJ, Roman PM. Adoption and implementation of medications in addiction treatment programs. *J Addict Med.* 2011;5(1):21–27.

15. Maryland Behavioral Health Administration. *Statewide standing order for pharmacy naloxone dispensing.* https://bha.health. maryland.gov/NALOXONE/Pages/Statewide-Standing-Order. aspx. Accessed August 29, 2018.

16. Troubled teen industry: help or harm? *Safe, Therapeutic & Appropriate Use of Residential Treatment (START).* 16 March 2015. http://astartforteens.org/. Accessed August 30, 2018.

17. US Government Accountability Office. *Residential treatment programs: Concerns regarding abuse and death in certain programs*

for troubled youth. 10 October 2017. https://www.gao.gov/products/GAO-08-146T. Accessed August 30, 2018.

18. US Government Accountability Office. *Residential treatment programs: Concerns regarding abuse and death in certain programs for troubled youth. 10 October 2017.* https://www.gao.gov/products/GAO-08-146T. Accessed August 30, 2018.

19. US Government Accountability Office. *Residential treatment programs: Concerns regarding abuse and death in certain programs for troubled youth.* 10 October 2017. https://www.gao.gov/products/GAO-08-146T. Accessed August 30, 2018.

20. Cabrera A, Weisfeldt S. Ex-patients, families say decades of abuse, fraud at Colorado facility ignored. *CNN.* 11 May 2014. https://www.cnn.com/2014/05/09/us/colorado-treatment-center-lawsuits/index.html. Accessed August 30, 2018.

21. Residential treatment programs for teens. *Federal Trade Commission.* July 2008. https://www.consumer.ftc.gov/articles/0185-residential-treatment-programs-teens. Accessed August 30, 2018.

22. Residential treatment programs for teens. *Federal Trade Commission.* July 2008. https://www.consumer.ftc.gov/articles/0185-residential-treatment-programs-teens. Accessed August 30, 2018.

Chapter 9

1. Bebinger M. Families choose empathy over "tough love" to rescue loved ones from opioids. *NPR.* 10 August 2018. https://www.npr.org/sections/health-shots/2018/08/10/636556573/families-choose-empathy-over-tough-love-to-rescue-loved-ones-from-opioids. Accessed August 31, 2018.

2. Sousares E. Why I abandoned tough love instead of my child. *Women's Day.* 1 July 2016. https://www.womansday.com/health-fitness/wellness/a55379/help-for-parents-of-drug-addicts. Accessed August 31, 2018.

3. "Unbroken Brain" explains why "tough" treatment doesn't help drug addicts. *NPR.* 7 July 2016. https://www.npr.org/sections/health-shots/2016/07/07/485087604/unbroken-brain-explains-why-tough-treatment-doesnt-help-drug-addicts. Accessed August 31, 2018.

Chapter 10

1. White, W. *Slaying the Dragon: The History of Addiction Treatment and Recovery in America.* 2nd ed. Bloomington, IL: Chestnut Health Systems; 2014.

2. Andersen KJ, Kallestrup CM. Rejected by A.A. *The New Republic.* 27 June 2018. https://newrepublic.com/article/149398/rejected-aa. Accessed August 30, 2018.

3. White, W. *Slaying the Dragon: The History of Addiction Treatment and Recovery in America.* 2nd ed. Bloomington, IL: Chestnut Health Systems; 2014.

4. White, W. *Slaying the Dragon: The History of Addiction Treatment and Recovery in America.* 2nd ed. Bloomington, IL: Chestnut Health Systems; 2014.

5. Stratman H, Aronberg D. Sober living homes and the regulation they need. *The Governing Institute.* 14 May 2018. http://www.governing.com/gov-institute/voices/col-regulation-sober-living-homes-recovery-residences-need.html. Accessed August 30, 2018.

6. Standards and certification program. *National Alliance for Recovery Residences.* 2016. http://narronline.org/affiliate-services/standards-and-certification-program/. Accessed August 30, 2018.

Chapter 11

1. Porter J, Jick H. Addiction rare in patients treated with narcotics. *N Engl J Med* 1980;302:123–123.

2. Hawkins D. How a short letter in a prestigious journal contributed to the opioid crisis. *The Washington Post.* 2 June 2017.

3. IQVIA. *Medicine Use and Spending in the U.S.* 19 April 2018. https://www.iqvia.com/institute/reports/medicine-use-and-spending-in-the-us review-of-2017-outlook to-2022. Accessed August 8, 2018.

4. Faulkner W. *Requiem for a Nun.* New York, NY: Random House, 1951.

5. Santayana G. *The Life of Reason: Reason in Common Sense.* Scribner's; 1905: 284.

6. Musto DF. *The American Disease: Origins of Narcotic Control.* 3rd ed. New York, NY: Oxford University Press; 1999: 69.

7. Courtwright DT. *Dark Paradise: A History of Opiate Addiction in America.* Cambridge, MA: Harvard University Press; 2001.

8. Courtwright DT. *Dark Paradise: A History of Opiate Addiction in America.* Cambridge: Harvard University Press; 2001.

9. Courtwright DT. *Dark Paradise: A History of Opiate Addiction in America.* Cambridge, MA: Harvard University Press; 2001.

10. Courtwright DT. *Dark Paradise: A History of Opiate Addiction in America.* Cambridge, MA: Harvard University Press; 2001.

11. Mrs. Winslow's soothing syrup: the baby killer. *Museum of Health Care Blog*. 28 July 2017. https://museumofhealthcare. wordpress.com/2017/07/28/mrs-winslows-soothing-syrup-the-baby-killer/. Accessed August 7, 2018. This patent remedy also contained alcohol.

12. Musto DF. *The American Disease: Origins of Narcotic Control*. 3rd ed. New York, NY: Oxford University Press; 1999: 21.

13. Miroff, N. From Teddy Roosevelt to Trump: the history of heroin and opioid addiction in the U.S. *The Washington Post*. 17 October 2017.

14. Musto DF. *The American Disease: Origins of Narcotic Control*. 3rd ed. New York, NY: Oxford University Press; 1999: 185.

15. Hilgers, L. Treat addiction like cancer. *The New York Times*. 19 May 2018.

16. Fernandez H, Libby T. *Heroin: its history, pharmacology, and treatment*. 2nd ed. Center City, MN: Hazelden; 2011: 156.

17. Musto DF. *The American Disease: Origins of Narcotic Control*. 3rd ed. New York, NY: Oxford University Press, 1999.

18. Nixon R. Special message to the Congress on drug abuse prevention and control. June 1971. *The American Presidency Project*. http://www.presidency.ucsb.edu/ws/?pid=3047. Accessed August 8, 2018.

19. Musto DF. *The American Disease: Origins of Narcotic Control*. 3rd ed. New York, NY: Oxford University Press; 1999: 125.

20. Institute of Medicine. *Relieving Pain in America: A Blueprint for Transforming Prevention, Care, Education, and Research*. Washington, DC: The National Academies Press; 2011: 69–71.

21. Mitka M. Experts debate widening use of opioid drugs for chronic nonmalignant pain. *JAMA*. 2003;289(18):2347–2348.

22. Van Zee A. The promotion and marketing of oxycontin: commercial triumph, public health tragedy. *Am J Public Health*. 2009;99(2):221–227.

23. Van Zee A. The promotion and marketing of OxyContin: commercial triumph, public health tragedy. *Am J Public Health*. 2009;99(2):221–227.

24. Chen JH, Humphreys K, Shah NH, Lembke A. Distribution of opioids by different types of Medicare prescribers. *JAMA Intern Med*. 2016;176(2):259–261.

25. Centers for Disease Control and Prevention. *Why Guidelines for Primary Care Providers?* https://www.cdc.gov/drugoverdose/pdf/guideline_infographic-a.pdf. Accessed August 21, 2018.

4

26. Wilkerson RG, Kim HK, Windsor TA, Mariniss D. The opioid epidemic in the United States. *Emerg Med Clin N Am.* 2016;34:1–23.
27. Quinones S. *Dreamland: The True Tale of America's Opiate Epidemic.* London: Bloomsbury; 2015: 94.
28. Institute of Medicine. *Relieving Pain in America: A Blueprint for Transforming Prevention, Care, Education, and Research.* Washington, DC: The National Academies Press; 2011: 145.
29. DeNoon D. The 10 most prescribed drugs. *WebMD.* 20 April 2011. https://www.webmd.com/drug-medication/news/20110420/the-10-most-prescribed-drugs#1. Accessed August 7, 2018.
30. Lembke A. *Drug Dealer, MD.* Baltimore, MD: Johns Hopkins University Press; 2016: 9.
31. Musto DF. *The American Disease: Origins of Narcotic Control.* 3rd ed. New York, NY: Oxford University Press; 1999: 140.
32. Ballantyne JC, Mao J. Opioid therapy for chronic pain. *N Engl J Med.* 2003;349(20):1943–1953.
33. Meier B, Petersen M. Sales of painkiller grew rapidly, but success brought a high cost. *The New York Times.* 5 March 2001.
34. Mitka M. Experts debate widening use of opioid drugs for chronic nonmalignant pain. *JAMA.* 2003;289(18):2347–2348.
35. Meier B. At Painkiller trouble spot, signs seen as alarming didn't alarm drug's maker. *The New York Times.* 10 December 2001.
36. Meier B. Overdoses of painkiller are linked to 282 deaths. *The New York Times.* 28 October 2001.
37. James C. Television review: A painkiller's double life as an illegal street drug. *The New York Times.* 12 December 2001.
38. James C. Television review: A painkiller's double life as an illegal street drug. *The New York Times.* 12 December 2001.
39. Meier B. Oxycontin prescribers face charges in fatal overdoses. *The New York Times.* 19 January 2002.
40. Thomas L. Maker of oxycontin reaches settlement with West Virginia. *The New York Times.* 6 November 2004.
41. Harder-to-break oxycontin pill wins approval. *Reuters.* 5 April 2010.
42. Alvarez L. Florida shutting "pill mill" clinics. *The New York Times.* 31 August 2011.
43. Houston T, Rich R. Opioid abuse and pain management. *Am Fam Physician.* 2012;86(7):600–602.
44. Dowell D, Haegerich TM, Chou R. CDC guideline for prescribing opioids for chronic pain—United States, 2016. *MMWR Recomm Rep.* 2016;65(1):1–49.

45. IQVIA. *Medicine Use and Spending in the U.S.* 19 April 2018. https://www.iqvia.com/institute/reports/medicine-use-and-spending-in-the-us-review-of-2017-outlook-to-2022. Accessed August 8, 2018.

46. Kliff S. "We started it": Atul Gawande on doctors' role in the opioid epidemic. *Vox*. 8 September 2017. https://www.vox.com/2017/9/8/16270370/atul-gawande-opioid-weeds. Accessed August 8, 2018.

47. Seelye K. Heroin in New England, more abundant and deadly. *The New York Times*. 18 July 2013.

48. Centers for Disease Control and Prevention. *Drug-Poisoning Deaths Involving Heroin: United States, 2000-2013*. March 2015. https://www.cdc.gov/nchs/data/databriefs/db190.pdf. Accessed August 8, 2018.

49. Centers for Disease Control and Prevention. *Vital Signs: Today's Heroin Epidemic*. 7 July 2015. https://www.cdc.gov/nchs/data/databriefs/db190.pdf. Accessed August 8, 2018.

50. Gupta S. Unintended consequences: why painkiller addicts turn to heroin. *CNN*. 2 June 2016. https://www.cnn.com/2014/08/29/health/gupta-unintended-consequences/index.html. Accessed August 8, 2018.

51. Buckley C. Young and suburban, and falling for heroin. *The New York Times*. 25 September 2009.

52. Quinones S. *Dreamland: The True Tale of America's Opiate Epidemic*. London: Bloomsbury Press; 2015.

53. Compton WM, Jones CM, Baldwin GT. Relationship between nonmedical prescription-opioid use and heroin use. *N Engl J Med*. 2016;374(2):154–163.

54. Paone D, Tuazon E, Kattan J, et al. Decrease in rate of opioid analgesic overdose deaths—Staten Island, New York City, 2011–2013. *MMWR Morb Mortal Wkly Rep*. 2015;64(18):491–494.

55. Rizzi N. Staten Island's fatal overdoses reached record high last year, data shows. *DNAinfo*. 3 March 2017. https://www.dnainfo.com/new-york/20170303/new-dorp/staten-island-fatal-overdoses-heroin-fentanyl-most-since-2000. Accessed August 9, 2018.

56. Jones T, Krzywicki, J, Jones N, et al. Nonpharmaceutical fentanyl-related deaths—multiple states, April 2005—March 2007. *MMWR Morb Mortal Wkly Rep*. 2008;57(29);793–796.

57. RI officials say dangerous opiate now in pill form. *Associated Press*. 13 October 2013.

58. Walker AK. Fentanyl-laced heroin killing Marylanders. *The Baltimore Sun.* 31 January 2014.

59. Drug Enforcement Agency. *2017 National Drug Threat Assessment.* 23 October 2017. https://www.dea.gov/docs/DIR-040-17_2017-NDTA.pdf. Accessed August 8, 2018.

60. Whelan J, Spegele, B. The Chinese connection fueling America's fentanyl crisis. *Wall Street Journal.* 23 June 2016.

61. Drug Enforcement Agency. *2017 National Drug Threat Assessment.* 23 October 2017. https://www.dea.gov/docs/DIR-040-17_2017-NDTA.pdf. Accessed August 8, 2018.

62. Prince had "exceedingly high" level of fentanyl in body when he died. *USA Today.* 26 March 2018.

63. Ellis R. Tom Petty died of accidental drug overdose, medical examiner says. *CNN.* 21 January 2018.

64. Du Bois WEB. *The Souls of Black Folk.* Chicago, IL: A.C. McClurg & Co; 1903.

65. Courtwright DT. *Dark Paradise: A History of Opiate Addiction in America.* Cambridge, MA: Harvard University Press; 2001.

66. Courtwright DT. *Dark Paradise: A History of Opiate Addiction in America.* Cambridge, MA: Harvard University Press; 2001.

67. Musto DF. *The American Disease: Origins of Narcotic Control.* 3rd ed. New York, NY: Oxford University Press; 1999: 17.

68. Musto DF. *The American Disease: Origins of Narcotic Control.* 3rd ed. New York, NY: Oxford University Press; 1999: 65.

69. Musto DF. *The American Disease: Origins of Narcotic Control.* 3rd ed. New York, NY: Oxford University Press; 1999.

70. Musto DF. *The American Disease: Origins of Narcotic Control.* 3rd ed. New York, NY: Oxford University Press; 1999.

71. Lurie J, Jula M. Now Republicans are blaming sanctuary cities for the opioid epidemic. *Mother Jones.* 15 February 2018.

72. Bump P. Maine governor says out-of-state drug dealers are impregnating 'young, white girl[s],' kind-of apologizes. *The Washington Post.* 8 January 2016.

Chapter 12

1. Tick H, Nielsen A, Pelletier KR, et al. Evidence-based nonpharmacologic strategies for comprehensive pain care. December 2017. https://www.north floridaspineand injurycenter.com/uploads/ Evidence-Based Nonpharmacologic Strategiesfor Compre hensive PainCare TheConsortium PainTask Force White Paper.pdf. Accessed August 11, 2018.

2. Thomas K, Ornstein C. Amid opioid crisis, insurers restrict pricey, less addictive painkillers. *The New York Times.* 17 September 2016.

3. Teegardin C. Medical board sending Georgia's doctors to opioid. *The Atlanta Journal-Constitution.* 10 August 2017. https://www.ajc.com/news/breaking-news/medical-board-sending-georgia-doctors-opioid-training/FQ3JvgidxsQd4hQNb9kZjK/. Accessed August 11, 2018.

4. Gottlieb S. In search of more rational prescribing. *U.S. Food and Drug Administration.* 4 April 2018. https://www.fda.gov/newsevents/speeches/ucm603651.htm. Accessed August 11, 2018.

5. Maryland takes one step forward and one step back against. *The Washington Post.* 18 May 2016.

6. Gottlieb S. In search of more rational prescribing. *US Food and Drug Administration.* 4 April 2018. https://www.fda.gov/newsevents/speeches/ucm603651.htm. Accessed August 11, 2018.

7. New opioid limits law passes. *Massachusetts Medical Society.* March 2016. http://www.massmed.org/News-and-Publications/Vital-Signs/New-Opioid-Limits-Law-Passes/#.W291-OhKheV. Accessed August 11, 2018.

8. Sanghavi D, Atlan A, Hane C, Bleicher P. *Health Affairs.* 18 December 2017. https://www.healthaffairs.org/do/10.1377/hblog20171215.681297/full/. Accessed August 11, 2018.

9. Johns Hopkins Bloomberg School of Public Health. *The opioid epidemic: from evidence to impact.* October 2017. https://www.jhsph.edu/events/2017/americas-opioid-epidemic/report/2017-JohnsHopkins-Opioid-digital.pdf. Accessed August, 12, 2018.

10. Johns Hopkins Bloomberg School of Public Health. *The opioid epidemic: from evidence to impact.* October 2017. https://www.jhsph.edu/events/2017/americas-opioid-epidemic/report/2017-JohnsHopkins-Opioid-digital.pdf. Accessed August, 12, 2018.

11. Weiner J, Bao Y, Meisel Z. *Prescription drug monitoring programs: evolution and evidence.* 8 June 2017. https://ldi.upenn.edu/brief/prescription-drug-monitoring-programs-evolution-and-evidence. Accessed August 12, 2018.

12. Department of Justice. *Drug enforcement administration collects record number of unused pills as part of its 14th prescription drug take back day.* 7 November 2017. https://www.justice.gov/opa/

pr/drug-enforcement-administration-collects-record-number-
unused-pills-part-its-14th-0. Accessed August 12, 2018.

13. Wynn RL. Opioid medication disposal programs: reviewing
    their effectiveness. *Wolters Kluwer.* 3 January 2017. http://www.
    wolterskluwercdi.com/blog/opioid-medication-disposal-
    programs-reviewing-their-effectiveness/. Accessed August
    12, 2018.

14. The FDA points out that most medications in wastewater are
    delivered by the human body, through excretion of drugs
    and their metabolites in urine and feces. Disposal of unused
    medicines: what you should know. *U.S. Food and Drugs
    Administration.* 25 July 2018. https://www.fda.gov/drugs/
    resourcesforyou/consumers/buyingusingmedicinesafely/
    ensuringsafeuseofmedicine/safedisposalofmedicines/
    ucm186187.htm. Accessed August 12, 2018.

15. Van Blokland H. 2 more former Insys employees plead guilty to
    kickback scheme. *KJZZ.* 12 July 2017. https://kjzz.org/content/
    503745/2-more-former-insys-employees-plead-guilty-kickback-
    scheme. Accessed August 12, 2018.

16. Centers for Disease Control and Prevention. *Clinical evidence
    review for the CDC guideline for prescribing opioids for chronic pain—
    United States, 2016.* 18 March 2016. https://stacks.cdc.gov/view/
    cdc/38026. Accessed August 12, 2018.

17. Dowell D, Haegerich TM, Chou R. *CDC Guideline for Prescribing
    Opioids for Chronic Pain—United States, 2016.* 15 March 2016.
    https://www.cdc.gov/mmwr/volumes/65/rr/rr6501e1.htm.
    Accessed August 12, 2018.

18. Gottlieb S. In search of more rational prescribing. *US Food
    and Drug Administration.* 4 April 2018. https://www.fda.gov/
    newsevents/speeches/ucm603651.htm. Accessed August
    11, 2018.

19. Baumgaertner E. FDA Did not intervene to curb risky fentanyl
    prescriptions. *The New York Times.* 2 August 2018.

20. @SGottliebFDA. We appreciate the #FDA advisory committee's
    discussion on the Risk Evaluation and Mitigation Strategy
    (REMS). https://twitter.com/SGottliebFDA/status/
    1025496746732998658. Posted August 3, 2018.

21. US Food and Drugs Administration. *FDA requests removal of
    Opana ER for risks related to abuse.* 8 June 2017. https://www.

fda.gov/NewsEvents/Newsroom/PressAnnouncements/
ucm562401.htm. Accessed August 12, 2018.

22. Peters PJ, Pontones P, Hoover KW, et al. HIV infection linked to injection use of oxymorphone in Indiana, 2014–2015. *N Engl J Med*. 2016;375(3):229–239.

23. National Academies of Sciences, Engineering, and Medicine. *Pain Management and the Opioid Epidemic: Balancing Societal and Individual Benefits and Risks of Prescription Opioid Use*. Washington, DC: The National Academies Press; 2017.

24. National Academies of Sciences, Engineering, and Medicine. *Pain Management and the Opioid Epidemic: Balancing Societal and Individual Benefits and Risks of Prescription Opioid Use*. Washington, DC: The National Academies Press; 2017.

25. National Academies of Science, Engineering, and Medicine. *The health effects of cannabis and cannabinoids: the current state of evidence and recommendations for research*. 12 January 2017. http://www.nationalacademies.org/hmd/Reports/2017/health-effects-of-cannabis-and-cannabinoids.aspx. Accessed September 1, 2018.

26. Bradford AC, Bradford WD, Abraham A, Bagwell Adams G. Association Between US state medical cannabis laws and opioid prescribing in the Medicare Part D population. *JAMA Intern Med*. 2018 May 1;178(5):667–672.

27. Bradford AC, Bradford WD. Medical marijuana laws may be associated with a decline in the number of prescriptions for Medicaid enrollees. *Health Aff* (Millwood). 2017 May 1;36(5):945–951.

28. Bachhuber MA, Saloner B, Cunningham CO, Barry CL. Medical cannabis laws and opioid analgesic overdose mortality in the United States, 1999–2010. *JAMA Intern Med*. 2014 Oct;174(10):1668–1673.

29. Livingston MD, Barnett TE, Delcher C, Wagenaar AC. Recreational cannabis legalization and opioid-related deaths in Colorado, 2000–2015. *Am J Public Health*. 2017 Nov;107(11):1827–1829.

30. Ingold J. More Coloradans died last year from drug overdoses than any year in the state's history: that shows how the opioid epidemic is changing. *Denver Post*. 4 April 2018. https://www.denverpost.com/2018/04/04/colorado-drug-overdoses-opioid-deaths-hit-high/. Accessed September 1, 2018.

31. Caputi TL, Humphreys K. Medical marijuana users are more likely to use prescription drugs medically and nonmedically. *J Addict Med.* 2018 Jul/Aug;12(4):295–299.

32. Olfson M, Wall MM, Liu SM, Blanco C. Cannabis use and risk of prescription opioid use disorder in the United States. *Am J Psychiatry.* 2018 Jan 1;175(1):47–53.

33. Open source: Could medical marijuana help address the opioid epidemic. *Hopkins Bloomberg Public Health Magazine.* Summer 2018. https://magazine.jhsph.edu/2018/open-source-could-medical-marijuana-help-address-opioid-epidemic. Accessed September 1, 2018.

34. Cerdá M, Sarvet AL, Wall M, et al. Medical marijuana laws and adolescent use of marijuana and other substances: alcohol, cigarettes, prescription drugs, and other illicit drugs. *Drug Alcohol Depend.* 2018 Feb 1;183:62–68.

35. Masters K. Chronic pain patients report struggles under tighter opioid regulations. *The Frederick News-Post.* 12 February 2018. https://www.fredericknewspost.com/news/health/hospitals_and_doctors/chronic-pain-patients-report-struggles-under-tighter-opioid-regulations/article_f6cdf517-ba94-59a6-8395-644ecccc77e2.html. Accessed August 12, 2018.

36. Kline T. #OpioidCrisis pain related suicides associated with forced tapers. *Medium.* 30 May 2018. https://medium.com/@ThomasKlineMD/opioidcrisis-pain-related-suicides-associated-with-forced-tapers-c68c79ecf84d. Accessed August 12, 2018.

37. Gottlieb S. In search of more rational prescribing. 4 April 2018. *U.S. Food and Drug Administration.* https://www.fda.gov/NewsEvents/Speeches/ucm603651.htm. Accessed August 11, 2018.

38. Human Resources and Services Administration. *Report of the Secretary's Advisory Committee on Infant Mortality (SACIM).* January 2013. http://www.hrsa.gov/advisorycommittees/mchbadvisory/InfantMortality/About/natlstrategyrecommendations.pdf. Accessed August 12, 2018.

39. Dube S, Felitti V, Dong M, Chapman D, Giles W, Anda R. Childhood abuse, neglect, and household dysfunction and the risk of illicit drug use: the Adverse Childhood Experiences study. *Pediatrics.* 2003;111(3):564–572.

40. Kellam S, Brown C, Poduska J, et al. Effects of a universal classroom behavior management program in first and second

grades on young adult behavioral, psychiatric, and social outcomes. *Drug Alcohol Depend.* 2008;95:S5–S28.

41. Kim BKE, Gloppen KM, Rhew IC, Oesterle S, Hawkins JD. Effects of the communities that care prevention system on youth reports of protective factors. *Prevention Science.* 2015;16(5):652–662.

42. Creating Communities that Care. *University of Washington.* October 2017. http://www.washington.edu/boundless/communities-that-care/. Accessed August 31, 2018.

43. Evidence-based practices resource center. *Substance Abuse and Mental Health Services Administration.* 3 April 2018. https://www.samhsa.gov/ebp-resource-center. Accessed August 21, 2018.

Chapter 13

1. Baltimore Substance Abuse Systems. *Steps to success: Baltimore drug and alcohol treatment outcomes study.* 2002. http://www.soros.org/initiatives/baltimore/articles_publications/publications/steps. Accessed April 30, 2018.

2. Substance Abuse Mental Health Services Administration. *Medications for opioid use disorder: for healthcare and addiction professionals, policymakers, patients, and families. Treatment improvement protocol (TIP) 63.* 18 February 2018. https://store.samhsa.gov/product/SMA18-5063FULLDOC. Accessed April 29, 2018.

3. National Institute on Drug Abuse. Effective treatment for opioid addiction. November 2016. https://www.drugabuse.gov/publications/effective-treatments-opioid-addiction/effective-treatments-opioid-addiction. Accessed August 31, 2018.

4. Centers for Disease Control and Prevention. Today's heroin epidemic. 7 July 2015. https://www.cdc.gov/vitalsigns/heroin/. Accessed August 31, 2018.

5. World Health Organization. *Guidelines for the Psychosocially Assisted Treatment of Opioid Dependence.* 2009. http://www.who.int/substance_abuse/publications/opioid_dependence_guidelines.pdf. Accessed August 31, 2018.

6. Schwartz RP, Gryczynski J, O'Grady KE, et al. Opioid agonist treatments and heroin overdose deaths in Baltimore, Maryland, 1995–2009. *Am J Public Health.* 2013;103(5):917–922.

7. Khazan O. How France cut heroin overdoses by 79 percent in 4 years. *The Atlantic.* 16 April 2018. https://www.theatlantic.com/health/archive/2018/04/

how-france-reduced-heroin-overdoses-by-79-in-four-years/
558023/. Accessed August 21, 2018.

8. D'Onofrio G, O'Connor PG, Pantalon M V., et al. Emergency
department–initiated buprenorphine/naloxone treatment for
opioid dependence. *JAMA*. 2015;313(16):1636.

9. George J. Why do so few docs have buprenorphine waivers?
Medpage Today. 14 February 2018. https://www.medpagetoday.
com/psychiatry/addictions/71169. Accessed September 1, 2018.

10. Knudsen HK. The supply of physicians waivered to prescribe
buprenorphine for opioid use disorders in the United States: a
state-level analysis. *J Stud Alcohol Drugs*. 2015 Jul;76(4):644–654.

11. American Correctional Association. *American Correctional
Association and American Society of Addiction Medicine release joint
policy statement on opioid use disorder treatment in the justice system*.
20 March 2018. http://www.aca.org/ACA_Prod_IMIS/DOCS/
ACA-ASAM%20Press%20Release%20and%20Joint%20Policy%20
Statement%203.20.18.pdf. Accessed August 12, 2018.

12. Green TC, Clarke J, Brinkley-Rubinstein L, et al.
Postincarceration fatal overdoses after implementing medications
for addiction treatment in a statewide correctional system. *JAMA
Psychiatry*. 2018;75(4):405–407.

13. Bernstein L. San Francisco will bring anti-addiction medication
to users on the streets. *The Washington Post*. 17 May 2018.

14. Reilly C, Arsenault S. Insurance coverage for substance use
disorder treatment impedes care. *The Pew Charitable Trusts*.
29 March 2017. http://www.pewtrusts.org/en/research-
and-analysis/articles/2017/03/29/insurance-coverage-for-
substance-use-disorder-treatment-impedes-care. Accessed
August 12, 2018.

15. Kaiser Family Foundation. *Total monthly Medicaid and CHIP
enrollment*. 2018. https://www.kff.org/health-reform/state-
indicator/total-monthly-medicaid-and-chip-enrollment/?current
Timeframe=0&sortModel=%7B%22colId%22:%22Location%22,%
22sort%22:%22asc%22%7D. Accessed August 12, 2018.

16. Kaiser Family Foundation. *Status of state action on the Medicaid
expansion decision*. 26 November 2018. https://www.kff.org/
health-reform/state-indicator/state-activity-around-expanding-
medicaid-under-the-affordable-care-act/?currentTimeframe=0&s
ortModel=%7B%22colId%22:%22Location%22,%22sort%22:%22a
sc%22%7D. Accessed December 9, 2018.

17. Scott D. Visualized: what Medicaid pays for addiction treatment meds, state by state. *Stat News*. https://www.statnews.com/2017/03/14/medicaid-addiction-treatment/. Accessed August 12, 2018.

18. Reilly C, Arsenault S. Insurance coverage for substance use disorder treatment impedes care. *The Pew Charitable Trusts*. 29 March 2017. http://www.pewtrusts.org/en/research-and-analysis/articles/2017/03/29/insurance-coverage-for-substance-use-disorder-treatment-impedes-care. Accessed August 12, 2018.

19. Grogan CM, Andrews C, Abraham A, et al. Survey highlights differences in Medicaid coverage for substance use treatment and opioid use disorder medications. *Health Affairs*. 2016;35(12):2289–2296.

20. Lurie J. Go to jail. Die from drug withdrawal. Welcome to the criminal justice system. *Mother Jones*. 5 February 2017. https://www.motherjones.com/politics/2017/02/opioid-withdrawal-jail-deaths/. Accessed August 12, 2018.

21. Krawczyk N, Picher CE, Feder KA, Saloner B. Only one in twenty justice-referred adults in specialty treatment for opioid use receive methadone or buprenorphine. *Health Affairs*. 2017;36(12):2046–2053.

22. Ann L. Schneiderman to help with insurance coverage for addiction and mental health issues. *WZOZ*. 11 May 2016. http://wzozfm.com/schneiderman-to-help-with-insurance-coverage-for-addiction-mental-health-issues/. Accessed August 12, 2018.

23. Sontag D. Addiction treatment with a dark side. *The New York Times*. 16 November 2013.

24. Segal D. City of addict entrepreneurs. *The New York Times*. 27 December 2017.

25. Segal D. A doctor with a phone and a mission. *The New York Times*. 27 December 2017.

26. Henry J. State shuts down Pasadena-based "Celebrity Rehab" center over death, repeated violations. *Pasadena Star News*. 4 August 2018. https://www.pasadenastarnews.com/2018/08/04/state-shuts-down-pasadena-based-celebrity-rehab-center-over-death-repeated-violations/. Accessed August 31, 2018.

27. Alvarez L. Haven for recovering addicts now profits from their relapses. *The New York Times*. 20 June 2017.

28. Kinder P. Not in my backyard phenomenon. *Encyclopaedia Britannica*. 14 June 2016. https://www.britannica.com/topic/Not-in-My-Backyard-Phenomenon. Accessed August 12, 2018.

29. Substance Abuse and Mental Health Services Administration. *Siting drug and alcohol treatment programs: legal challenges to the NIMBY syndrome.* 1995. http://adaiclearinghouse.org/downloads/tap-14-siting-drug-and-alcohol-treatment-programs-legal-challenges-to-the-nimby-syndrome-104.pdf. Accessed August 12, 2018.

30. Substance Abuse and Mental Health Services Administration. *Siting drug and alcohol treatment programs: legal challenges to the NIMBY syndrome.* 1995. http://adaiclearinghouse.org/downloads/tap-14-siting-drug-and-alcohol-treatment-programs-legal-challenges-to-the-nimby-syndrome-104.pdf. Accessed August 12, 2018.

31. Furr-Holden CD, Milam AJ, Nesoff ED, et al. Not in my back yard: a comparative analysis of crime around publicly funded drug treatment centers, liquor stores, convenience stores, and corner stores in one mid-Atlantic city. *J Stud Alcohol Drugs.* 2016;77(1):17–24.

32. Treatment here, not Timbuktu. Editorial. *Baltimore Sun.* 11 July 2017.

33. Americans with Disabilities Act, 42 USC § 202 (1990).

34. Substance Abuse and Mental Health Services Administration. *Siting drug and alcohol treatment programs: legal challenges to the NIMBY syndrome.* 1995. http://adaiclearinghouse.org/downloads/tap-14-siting-drug-and-alcohol-treatment-programs-legal-challenges-to-the-nimby-syndrome-104.pdf. Accessed August 12, 2018.

35. Cherkis J. Dying to be free. *The Huffington Post.* 28 January 2015. http://projects.huffingtonpost.com/dying-to-be-free-heroin-treatment. Accessed August 12, 2018.

36. National Center for Health Statistics. *Drug Overdose Mortality by State.* 10 January 2018. https://www.cdc.gov/nchs/pressroom/sosmap/drug_poisoning_mortality/drug_poisoning.htm. August 12, 2018.

37. Kaiser Family Foundation. *Opioid Overdose Death Rates and All Drug Overdose Death Rates per 100,000 Population (Age-Adjusted).* 2018. https://www.kff.org/other/state-indicator/opioid-overdose-death-rates/? current

Timeframe= 0&sortModel=%7B%22 colId%22:%22Opioid%20
Overdose%20Death%20 Rate%20(Age-Adjusted)%22,%
22sort%22:%22desc%22%7D. Accessed August 15, 2018.

38. My neighborhood, the methadone clinic: part I. *Brooklyn Reader*. 2
April 2014. https://www.bkreader.com /2014/04/my-neighbor-
the-methadone- clinic-part-i/. Accessed August 12, 2018.

39. The drug free moms and babies project. *West Virginia Perinatal
Partnership*. https://wvperinatal.org/ initiatives/substance-
use-during-pregnancy/ drug-free-moms-and- babies-project/.
Accessed August 13, 2018.

40. Hall MT, Wilfong J, Huebner RA, Posze L, Willauer
T. Medication-Assisted Treatment Improves Child Permanency
Outcomes for Opioid-Using Families in the Child Welfare
System. *J Subst Abuse Treat*. 2016 Dec;71:63–67.

41. Vestal C. Support grows for civil commitment of opioid
users. *Stateline*. 15 June 2017. http://www.pewtrusts.org/en/
research-and-analysis/blogs/stateline/2017/06/15/support-
grows-for-civil-commitment-of-opioid-users. Accessed August
21, 2018.

42. Stout M, Freyer FJ, McCluskey PD. Legislators reach deal on
opioids, but not on health care by end of session. *The Boston
Globe*. 31 July 2018.

43. Mings E, Cramp J. Best practices in peer support. *Addictions &
Mental Health Ontario*. 2014. http://eenet.ca/sites/default/files/
wp-content/uploads/2014/08/Best-Practices-PeerSupport-Final-
Report-2014.pdf. Accessed August 21, 2018.

44. Behavioral Health System Baltimore. *Threshold to recovery*. http://
www.bhsbaltimore.org/threshold-to-recovery/. Accessed
August 14, 2018.

45. Padgett DK, Stanhope V, Henwood BF, Stefancic A. Substance
use outcomes among homeless clients with serious mental
illness: comparing housing first with treatment first programs.
Community Ment Health J. 2011;47(2):227–232.

46. Larimer M, Malone D, Garner M, et al. Health care and public
service use and costs before and after provision of housing for
chronically homeless persons with severe alcohol problems.
JAMA. 2009;301(13):1349.

47. Marshall T, Goldberg R, Braude L, et al. Supported
employment: assessing the evidence. *Psychiatr Serv*.
2014;65(1):16–23.

Chapter 14

1. Harm Reduction Coalition. Principles of harm reduction. http://harmreduction.org/about-us/principles-of-harm-reduction/. Accessed August 14, 2018.

2. Harm Reduction Coalition. Principles of harm reduction. http://harmreduction.org/about-us/principles-of-harm-reduction/. Accessed August 14, 2018.

3. Harm Reduction Coalition. Principles of harm reduction. http://harmreduction.org/about-us/principles-of-harm-reduction/. Accessed August 14, 2018.

4. Hawk K, Vaca F, Onofrio G. Reducing fatal opioid overdose: prevention, treatment and harm reduction strategies. *Yale J Biol Med*. 2015;88(3):235–245.

5. Hawk K, Vaca F, Onofrio G. Reducing fatal opioid overdose: prevention, treatment and harm reduction strategies. *Yale J Biol Med*. 2015;88(3):235–245.

6. Castillo T. Harm reduction strategies for the opioid crisis. *N C Med J*. 2018;79(3):192–194.

7. Walley A, Xuan Z, Hackman H, et al. Opioid overdose rates and implementation of overdose education and nasal naloxone distribution in Massachusetts: interrupted time series analysis. *BMJ*. 2013;346:f174.

8. Mahoney K. FDA supports greater access to naloxone to help reduce opioid overdose deaths. *FDA Voice*. 10 August 2016. https://blogs.fda.gov/fdavoice/index.php/2016/08/fda-supports-greater-access-to-naloxone-to-help-reduce-opioid-overdose-deaths/. Accessed August 15, 2018.

9. Naloxone overdose prevention laws. *PDAPS (Prescription Drug Abuse Policy System)*. 1 July 2017. http://pdaps.org/datasets/laws-regulating-administration-of-naloxone-1501695139. Accessed August 24, 2018.

10. Hawk K, Vaca F, Onofrio G. Reducing fatal opioid overdose: prevention, treatment and harm reduction strategies. *Yale J Biol Med*. 2015;88(3):235–245.

11. Hawk K, Vaca F, Onofrio G. Reducing fatal opioid overdose: prevention, treatment and harm reduction strategies. *Yale J Biol Med*. 2015;88(3):235–245.

12. See, e.g., Hagan H, McGough JP, Thiede H, Hopkins S, Duchin J, Alexander ER. Reduced injection frequency and increased entry and retention in drug treatment associated with needle-exchange

participation in Seattle drug injectors. *J Subst Abuse Treat.* 2000;19(3):247–252.

13. Broadhead R, van Hulst Y, Heckathorn D. The impact of a needle exchange's closure. *Public Health Rep.* 1999;114(5):439–447. http://www.ncbi.nlm.nih.gov/pubmed/10590766. Accessed August 15, 2018.

14. Ksobiech K. Return rates for needle exchange programs: a common criticism answered. *Harm Reduct J.* 2004;1(1):2.

15. Tookes HE, Kral AH, Wenger LD, et al. A comparison of syringe disposal practices among injection drug users in a city with versus a city without needle and syringe programs. *Drug Alcohol Depend.* 2012;123(1–3):255–259.

16. Centers for Disease Control and Prevention. *Reducing harms from injection drug use & opioid use disorder with syringe services program.* August 2017. https://www.cdc.gov/hiv/pdf/risk/cdchiv-fs-syringe-services.pdf. Accessed August 24, 2018.

17. Freese A. Burlington to ease access to opioid addiction medication. *Seven Days.* 13 June 2018. https://www.sevendaysvt.com/vermont/burlington-to-ease-access-to-opioid-addiction-medication/Content?oid=16884183. Accessed August 15, 2018.

18. Bluthenthal RN, Ridgeway G, Schell T, Anderson R, Flynn NM, Kral AH. Examination of the association between syringe exchange program (SEP) dispensation policy and SEP client-level syringe coverage among injection drug users. *Addiction.* 2007;102(4):638–646.

19. Sherman S, Green T. Fentanyl Overdose Reduction Checking Analysis Study (FORECAST). 6 February 2018. http://americanhealth.jhu.edu/sites/default/files/inline-files/Fentanyl_Executive_Summary_032018.pdf. Accessed August 22, 2018.

20. Sherman S, Green T. Fentanyl Overdose Reduction Checking Analysis Study (FORECAST). 6 February 2018. http://americanhealth.jhu.edu/sites/default/files/inline-files/Fentanyl_Executive_Summary_032018.pdf. Accessed August 22, 2018.

21. Sherman S, Green T. Fentanyl Overdose Reduction Checking Analysis Study (FORECAST). 6 February 2018. http://americanhealth.jhu.edu/sites/default/files/inline-files/Fentanyl_Executive_Summary_032018.pdf. Accessed August 22, 2018.

22. Sherman S, Green T. Fentanyl Overdose Reduction Checking Analysis Study (FORECAST). 6 February 2018. http://americanhealth.jhu.edu/sites/default/files/inline-files/Fentanyl_Executive_Summary_032018.pdf. Accessed August 22, 2018.

23. Sherman S, Green T. Fentanyl Overdose Reduction Checking Analysis Study (FORECAST). 6 February 2018. http://americanhealth.jhu.edu/sites/default/files/inline-files/Fentanyl_Executive_Summary_032018.pdf. Accessed August 22, 2018.

24. Sherman S, Hunter K, Rouhani S. *Safe Drug Consumption Spaces: A Strategy for Baltimore City*. February 2017. https://www.abell.org/sites/default/files/files/Safe%20Drug%20Consumption%20Spaces%20final print%2072517.pdf. Accessed August 15, 2018.

25. Rosenstein R. Fight drug abuse, don't subsidize it. *The New York Times*. 27 August 2018. https://www.nytimes.com/2018/08/27/opinion/opioids-heroin-injection-sites.html. Accessed August 29, 2018.

26. Marshall BD, Milloy MJ, Wood E, Montaner JS, Kerr T. Reduction in overdose mortality after the opening of North America's first medically supervised safer injecting facility: a retrospective population-based study. *Lancet*. 2011;377(9775):1429–1437.

27. DeBeck K, Kerr T, Bird L, et al. Injection drug use cessation and use of North America's first medically supervised safer injecting facility. *Drug Alcohol Depend*. 2011;113(2–3):172–176.

28. Small W, Van Borek N, Fairbairn N, Wood E, Kerr T. Access to health and social services for IDU: the impact of a medically supervised injection facility. *Drug Alcohol Rev*. 2009;28(4):341–346.

29. Wood E, Kerr T, Small W, et al. Changes in public order after the opening of a medically supervised safer injecting facility for illicit injection drug users. *CMAJ*. 2004;171(7):731–734.

30. May T, Bennett T, Holloway K. The impact of medically supervised injection centres on drug-related harms: A meta-analysis. *Int J Drug Policy*. 2018;59:98–107. This article was retracted in September 2018 on the basis of methodological flaws. https://www.ijdp.org/article/S0955-3959(18)30180-4/fulltext. Accessed September 29, 2018.

31. Peterson DJ. Association of Schools & Programs of Public Health. Letter to Editor of the New York Times. 31 August 2018.

32. Barry CL, Sherman SG, McGinty EE. Language matters in combating the opioid epidemic: safe consumption sites versus overdose prevention sites. *Am J Public Health.* 2018;108(9):1157–1159.

33. Hunt N. A review of the evidence-base for harm reduction approaches to drug use. *Forward Thinking on Drugs.* 2003. http:// www.neilhunt.org/pdf/2003-evidence-base-for-hr-hunt-et-al.pdf. Accessed August 15, 2018.

34. Mattson CL, O'Donnell J, Kariisa M, Seth P, Scholl L, Gladden RM. Opportunities to prevent overdose deaths involving prescription and illlicit opioids, 11 states, July 2016–June 2017. *MMWR Morb Mortal Wkly Rep.* 2018;67(34):945–951.

35. McGinty E, Barry C, Stone E, et al. Public support for safe consumption sites and syringe services programs to combat the opioid epidemic. *Prev Med.* 2018;111:73–77.

36. Raymond D. Hitting Bottom on the politics of punishment: needle exchange and the costs of inaction. *Medium.* 8 April 2015. https://medium.com/@ danielraymond/hitting-bottom-on-the-politics-of-punishment-needle-exchange-and-the-costs-of-inaction-d83eadaa0790. Accessed August 15, 2018.

Chapter 15

1. Massing M. *The Fix.* New York, NY: Simon & Shuster; 1988: 97.

2. Turnaround on drugs? *The New York Times.* 5 September 1972.

3. Massing M. *The Fix.* New York, NY: Simon & Shuster; 1998: 129.

4. Massing M. *The Fix.* New York, NY: Simon & Shuster; 1998: 126.

5. Massing M. *The Fix.* New York, NY: Simon & Shuster; 1998: 129.

6. Massing M. *The Fix.* New York, NY: Simon & Shuster; 1998: 160.

7. Massing M. *The Fix.* New York, NY: Simon & Shuster; 1998: 184.

8. Travis J, Western B, Redburn S, et al. *The Growth of Incarceration in the United States.* Washington, DC: National Academies Press; 2014.

9. Massing M. *The Fix.* New York, NY: Simon & Shuster; 1998: 4.

10. The war on drugs, explained. *Vox.* 8 May 2016. https://www. vox.com/cards/war-on-drugs-marijuana-cocaine-heroin-meth/war-on-drugs-success-failure-working. Accessed August 15, 2018.

11. Polomarkakis KA. Drug law enforcement revisited: the "war" against the war on drugs. *J Drug Issues.* 2017;47(3):396–404.

12. The Pew Charitable Trusts. *More imprisonment does not reduce state drug problems*. March 2018. http://www.pewtrusts.org/-/media/assets/2018/03/pspp_more_imprisonment_does_not_reduce_state_drug_problems.pdf. Accessed August 15, 2018.

13. Mazerolle L, Soole D, Rombouts S. Drug law enforcement. *Police Q*. 2007;10(2):115–153.

14. Shultz P, Aspe P. The failed war on drugs. *The New York Times*. 31 December 2017.

15. DeBeck K, Cheng T, Montaner JS, et al. HIV and the criminalisation of drug use among people who inject drugs: a systematic review. *Lancet HIV*. 2017;4(8):e357–e374.

16. Massing M. *The Fix*. New York, NY: Simon & Shuster; 1988: 9.

17. Travis J, Western B, Redburn S, et al. *The Growth of Incarceration in the United States*. Washington, DC: National Academies Press; 2014.

18. Travis J, Western B, Redburn S, et al. *The Growth of Incarceration in the United States*. Washington, DC: National Academies Press; 2014.

19. Alexander M. *The New Jim Crow*. New York, NY: The New Press; 2010.

20. Alexander M. *The New Jim Crow*. New York, NY: The New Press; 2010.

21. Travis J, Western B, Redburn S, et al. *The Growth of Incarceration in the United States*. Washington, DC: National Academies Press; 2014.

22. Alexander M. *The New Jim Crow*. New York, NY: The New Press; 2010.

23. Travis J, Western B, Redburn S, et al. *The Growth of Incarceration in the United States*. Washington, DC: National Academies Press; 2014.

24. Goldensohn R. They shared drugs. Someone died. Does that make them killers? *The New York Times*. 25 May 2018.

25. Sanger D and Haberman M. Trump praises Duterte for Philippine drug crackdown in call transcript. *The New York Times*. 23 May 2017.

26. Berehulak D. "They are slaughtering us like animals.' *The New York Times*. 7 December 2016.

27. The Police Executive Research Forum. *Ten standards of care: policing and the opioid crisis*. April 2018. http://americanhealth.jhu.edu/sites/default/files/inline-files/

PolicingOpioidCrisis_LONG_final_0.pdf. Accessed August 20, 2018.

28. New York City Department of Health and Mental Hygiene. *RxStat: Opioid analgesic use and misuse in New York City*. September 2013. https://www1.nyc.gov/assets/home/downloads/ pdf/press-releases/2013/rx_stat_september_2013_report.pdf. Accessed August 15, 2018.

29. Brinkley-Rubinstein L, Zaller N, Martino S, et al. Criminal justice continuum for opioid users at risk of overdose. *Addict Behav*. 2018;86:104–110.

30. Mazerolle L, Soole D, Rombouts S. Drug law enforcement. *Police Q*. 2007;10(2):115–153.

31. The Pew Charitable Trusts. *More imprisonment does not reduce state drug problems*. March 2018. http://www.pewtrusts. org/-/media/assets/2018/03/pspp_more_imprisonment_ does_not_reduce_state_drug_problems.pdf. Accessed August 15, 2018.

32. Krawczyk N, Picher CE, Feder KA, Saloner B. Only one In twenty justice-referred adults In specialty treatment for opioid use receive methadone or buprenorphine. *Health Aff*. 2017;36(12):2046–2053.

33. Lurie J. Go to jail. Die from drug withdrawal. Welcome to the criminal justice system. *Mother Jones*. 5 February 2017. https:// www.motherjones.com/politics/2017/02/opioid-withdrawal- jail-deaths/. Accessed August 12, 2018.

34. Binswanger IA, Stern MF, Deyo RA, et al. Release from prison—a high risk of death for former inmates. *N Engl J Med*. 2007;356(2):157–165.

35. Green TC, Clarke J, Brinkley-Rubinstein L, et al. Postincarceration fatal overdoses after implementing medications for addiction treatment in a statewide correctional system. *JAMA Psychiatry*. 2018;75(4):405–407.

36. Farrell-MacDonald S, MacSwain MA, Cheverie M, Tiesmaki M, Fischer B. Impact of methadone maintenance treatment on women offenders' post-release recidivism. *Eur Addict Res*. 2014;20(4):192–199.

37. The President's Commission on Combating Drug Addiction and the Opioid Crisis. *Final Report*. 1 November 2017. https://www. whitehouse.gov/sites/whitehouse.gov/files/images/Final_ Report_Draft_11-15-2017.pdf. Accessed August 31, 2018.

38. American Correctional Association and American Society of Addiction Medicine release joint policy statement on opioid use disorder treatment in the justice system. 20 March 2018. https://www.aca.org/ACA_Prod_IMIS/DOCS/ACA-ASAM%20Press%20Release%20and%20Joint%20Policy%20Statement%203.20.18.pdf. Accessed August 31, 2018.

39. Monico LB, Mitchell SG, Gryczynski J. Prior experience with non-prescribed buprenorphine: role in treatment entry and retention. *J Subst Abuse Treat*. 2015;57:57–62.

40. Lofwall MR, Havens JR. Inability to access buprenorphine treatment as a risk factor for using diverted buprenorphine. *Drug Alcohol Depend*. 2012;126(3):379–383.

41. Freese A. Burlington to ease access to opioid addiction medication. *Seven Days*. 13 June 2018. https://www.sevendaysvt.com/vermont/burlington-to-ease-access-to-opioid-addiction-medication/Content?oid=16884183. Accessed August 29, 2018.

42. Marimow A. To cut prison drug smuggling, Maryland is restricting inmates' access to books. *The Washington Post*. 27 May 2018.

43. Washburn L. Drug treatment in NJ's jails helps break cycle of crime and addiction. NorthJersey.com. 6 August 2018. https://www.northjersey.com/story/news/2018/08/06/drug-treatment-nj-jails-helps-break-cycle-crime-and-addiction/913078002/. Accessed August 31, 2018.

44. Freyer F. US investigating treatment of addicted prisoners in Mass. *The Boston Globe*. 29 March 2018.

45. Walters Q. Judge rules Essex County Jail must give man methadone for Opioid addiction. 27 November 2018. https://www.wbur.org/commonhealth/2018/11/27/methadone-jail-massachusetts-geoffrey-pesce. Accessed December 9, 2018.

46. Frayer L. In Portugal, drug use is treated as a medical issue, not a crime. *NPR*. 18 April 2017. https://www.npr.org/sections/parallels/2017/04/18/524380027/in-portugal-drug-use-is-treated-as-a-medical-issue-not-a-crime. Accessed August 15, 2018.

47. Hall A, Coyne C. The militarization of U.S. domestic policing. *Indep Rev*. 2013;17(4):485–499.

48. Frayer L. In Portugal, drug use is treated as a medical issue, not a crime. *NPR*. 18 April 2017. https://www.npr.org/sections/parallels/2017/04/18/524380027/

in-portugal-drug-use-is-treated-as-a-medical-issue-not-a-crime. Accessed August 15, 2018.

49. Auriacombe M, Fatséas M, Dubernet J, Daulouède J-P, Tignol J. French field experience with Buprenorphine. *Am J Addict.* 2004;13(Suppl 1):S17–S28.

Chapter 16

1. Slavova S, O'Brien D, Creppage K, et al. Drug overdose deaths: let's get specific. *Public Health Rep.* 2015;130(4):339–342.

2. Horon IL, Singal P, Fowler DR, Sharfstein JM. Standard death certificates versus enhanced surveillance to identify heroin overdose-related deaths. *Am J Public Health.* 2018;108(6):777–781.

3. Substance Abuse and Mental Health Data Archive. *Drug Abuse Warning Network (DAWN).* https://www.datafiles.samhsa.gov/study-series/drug-abuse-warning-network-dawn-nid13516. Accessed August 15, 2018.

4. Jiang Y, Mcdonald J, Wilson M, et al. Rhode Island unintentional drug overdose death trends and ranking-office of the state medical examiners database. *R I Med J.* February 2018. http://www.rimed.org/rimedicaljournal/2018/02/2018-02-33-health-jiang.pdf. Accessed August 15, 2018.

5. Yang L, Wong L, Grivel M, Hasin D. Stigma and substance use disorders: an international phenomenon. *Curr Opin Psychiatry.* 2017;30(5):378–388.

6. Morgan R. A controversial study suggests anti-overdose med naloxone increases reckless opioid use. *CNBC.* 14 March 2018. https://www.cnbc.com/2018/03/14/study-suggests-anti-overdose-med-narcan-increases-reckless-opioid-use.html. Accessed August 20, 2018.

7. Walley A, Xuan Z, Hackman H, et al. Opioid overdose rates and implementation of overdose education and nasal naloxone distribution in Massachusetts: interrupted time series analysis. *BMJ.* 2013;346:f174.

8. Collins FS, Koroshetz WJ, Volkow ND. Helping to end addiction over the long-term. *JAMA.* 2018;320(2):129.

9. Sherman S, Green T. *Fentanyl Overdose Reduction Checking Analysis Study (FORECAST).* February 2018. http://americanhealth.jhu.edu/assets/pdfs/FORECAST_Summary_Report.pdf. Accessed August 20, 2018.

10. Sharfstein JM. The opioid crisis: from research to practice. *Milbank Q.* 2017 Mar;95(1):24–27.

11. Morris ZS, Wooding S, Grant J. The answer is 17 years, what is the question: understanding time lags in translational research. *J R Soc Med.* 2011;104(12):510–520.

12. Sharfstein J. *The Public Health Crisis Survival Guide.* New York, NY: Oxford University Press; 2018: 52.

Chapter 17

1. The Police Executive Research Forum. *Ten standards of care: policing and the opioid crisis.* April 2018. http://americanhealth.jhu.edu/sites/default/files/inline-files/PolicingOpioidCrisis_LONG_final_0.pdf. Accessed August 20, 2018.

2. Trone J. David and Goliath. *Vera Institute of Justice.* 2018. https://www.vera.org/the-human-toll-of-jail/david-and-goliath. Accessed August 20, 2018.

3. City of Manchester, New Hampshire. *Safe Station.* 2018. https://www.manchesternh.gov/Departments/Fire/Safe-Station. Accessed August 20, 2018.

4. Seelye K. In annual speech, Vermont governor shifts focus to drug abuse. *The New York Times.* 8 January 2014.

5. Text of Ohio Gov. John Kasich's 2017 State of the State address. *Akron Beacon Journal.* 4 April 2017. https://www.ohio.com/akron/news/text-of-ohio-gov-john-kasich-s-2017-state-of-the-state-address. Accessed August 20, 2018.

6. Kaiser Family Foundation. *Medicaid's role in addressing the opioid epidemic.* 27 February 2018. https://www.kff.org/infographic/medicaids-role-in-addressing-opioid-epidemic/. Accessed August 20, 2018.

7. Saloner B, Levin J, Chang HY. Changes in buprenorphine-naloxone and opioid pain reliever prescriptions after the Affordable Care Act Medicaid expansion. *JAMA Network Open.* 2018;1(4):e181588.

8. Ingles J. Gov. Kasich credits Medicaid expansion for helping Ohio fight drug abuse problem. *Statehouse.* 4 Jan 2017. http://www.statenews.org/post/gova-kasich-credits-medicaid-expansion-helping-ohio-fight-drug-abuse-problem. Accessed August 20, 2018. He later warned: "Now at some point, I will be gone and it will be very easy to cut the programs for people

who need help. Don't let it happen folks." Ingles J. Kasich warns fellow Republicans against undercutting Ohio's Medicaid expansion. *WOSU*. 2 April 2018. http://radio.wosu.org/post/ kasich-warns-fellow-republicans-against-undercutting-ohios-medicaid-expansion#stream/0. Accessed August 20, 2018.

9. In July 2018, a team of experts from Johns Hopkins University provided a set of recommendations to the State of Delaware on how to improve its treatment system. See Bloomberg American Health Initiative. *A blueprint for transforming opioid use disorder treatment in Delaware*. July 2018. http://dhss.delaware.gov/dhss/ files/johnshopkinsrep.pdf. Accessed August 20, 2018.

10. Arditi L. Overdose epidemic: Hasbro CEO, wife say R.I. hospital failed their son. *Providence Journal*. 9 March 2016. http://www. providencejournal.com/news/20160309/overdose-epidemic-hasbro-ceo-wife-say-ri-hospital-failed-their-son. Accessed August 21, 2018.

11. Rhode Island Department of Health. *Levels of care for Rhode Island emergency departments and hospitals for treating overdose and opioid use disorder*. March 2017. http://health.ri.gov/publications/ guides/LevelsOfCareForTreatingOverdoseAndOpioidUseDisor der.pdf. Accessed August 21, 2018.

12. Clark CB, Hendricks PS, Lane PS, Trent L, Cropsey KL. Methadone maintenance treatment may improve completion rates and delay opioid relapse for opioid dependent individuals under community corrections supervision. *Addict Behav*. 2014;39(12):1736–1740.

13. Farrell-MacDonald S, MacSwain MA, Cheverie M, Tiesmaki M, Fischer B. Impact of methadone maintenance treatment on women offenders' post-release recidivism. *Eur Addict Res*. 2014;20(4):192–199.

14. Krawczyk N, Picher C, Feder K, Saloner B. Only one in twenty justice-referred adults in specialty treatment for opioid use receive methadone or buprenorphine. *Health Aff*. 2017;36(12):2046–2053.

15. *Rhode Island's strategic plan on addiction and overdose*. 4 November 2015. http://www.health.ri.gov/news/temp/RhodeIslandsS trategicPlanOnAddictionAndOverdose.pdf. Accessed August 21, 2018.

16. Green TC, Clarke J, Brinkley-Rubinstein L, et al. Postincarceration fatal overdoses after implementing medications

for addiction treatment in a statewide correctional system. *JAMA Psychiatry*. 2018;75(4):405.

17. Massachusetts Department of Public Health. *An assessment of fatal and nonfatal opioid overdoses in Massachusetts (2011–2015)*. August 2017. https://www.mass.gov/files/documents/2017/08/31/legislative-report-chapter-55-aug-2017.pdf. Accessed August 21, 2018.

18. Larochelle M, Bernson D, Land T, et al. Medication for opioid use disorder after nonfatal opioid overdose and association with mortality. *Ann Intern Med*. 2018;169(3):137.

19. Lawmakers send opioid bill to Baker's desk. *WBUR*. 1 August 2018. http://www.wbur.org/commonhealth/2018/08/01/opioid-legislation-to-governor. Accessed August 21, 2018.

20. Seelye K. In annual speech, Vermont governor shifts focus to drug abuse. *The New York Times*. 8 January 2014.

21. Roubein R. Warren, Cummings seek $100B to fight opioid epidemic. *The Hill*. 18 April 2018.

22. Sanger D, Haberman M. Trump praises Duterte for Philippine drug crackdown in call transcript. *The New York Times*. 23 May 2017.

23. Shultz G, Aspe P. The failed war on drugs. *The New York Times*. 31 December 2017.

INDEX